CASSEY HO'S
HOT BODY
YEAR-ROUND

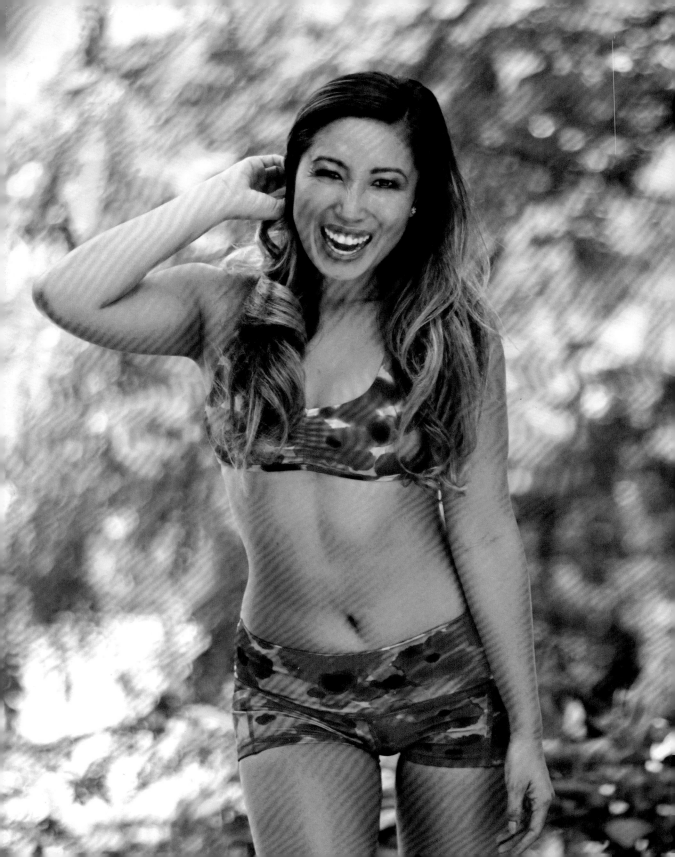

CASSEY HO'S HOT BODY YEAR-ROUND

THE POP PILATES PLAN TO GET SLIM, EAT CLEAN, AND LIVE HAPPY THROUGH EVERY SEASON

CASSEY HO

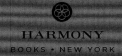

HARMONY
BOOKS · NEW YORK

Copyright © 2015 by Cassey Ho and oGorgeous Inc.

All rights reserved.
Published in the United States by Harmony Books, an imprint of the Crown Publishing Group, a
division of Random House LLC, a Penguin Random House Company, New York.
www.crownpublishing.com

Harmony Books is a registered trademark, and the Circle colophon is a trademark
of Random House LLC.

Library of Congress Cataloging-in-Publication Data
Ho, Cassey.
Cassey Ho's Hot Body Year-Round / by Cassey Ho.
pages cm
1. Pilates method. 2. Reducing exercises. 3. Reducing diets.
I. Title.
RA781.4.H6   2015
613.7'192—dc23
2014021074

ISBN 978-0-8041-3904-5
eBook ISBN 978-0-8041-3905-2

Printed in China

Book design by Jennifer K. Beal Davis
Photographs © 2015 by Sam Livits
Photographs © 2015 by David Kim
Cover design by Gabriel Levine
Cover photography by Mike Rosenthal
Cover illustrations: Shuttterstock/Alexander Tihonov (background);
Shuttterstock/Picsfive (vintage note papers);
Shuttterstock/Mtkang (photo frame);
Shuttterstock/Lainea (masking tapes);
Shuttterstock/jannoon028 (white notebook paper)

1 3 5 7 9 10 8 6 4 2

First Edition

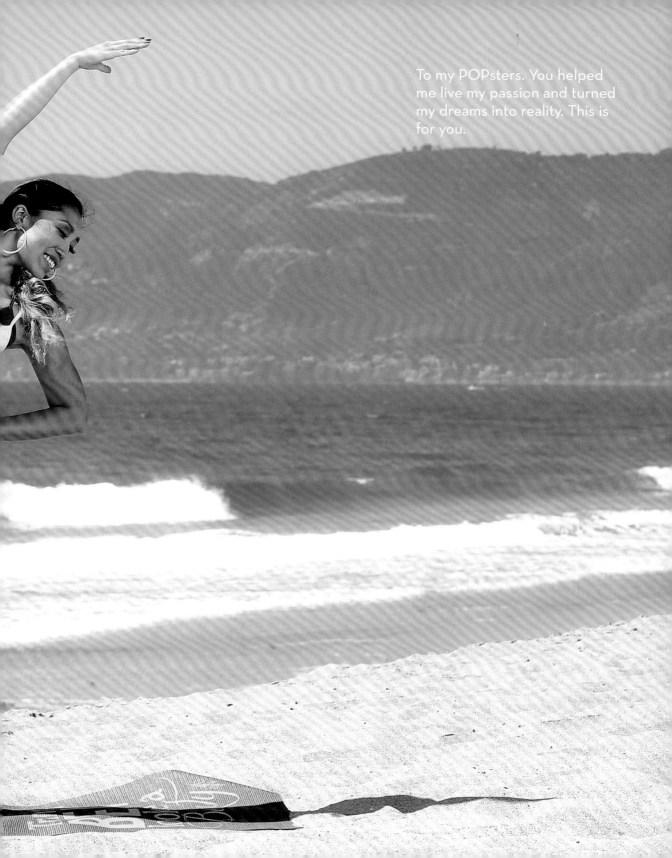

To my POPsters. You helped me live my passion and turned my dreams into reality. This is for you.

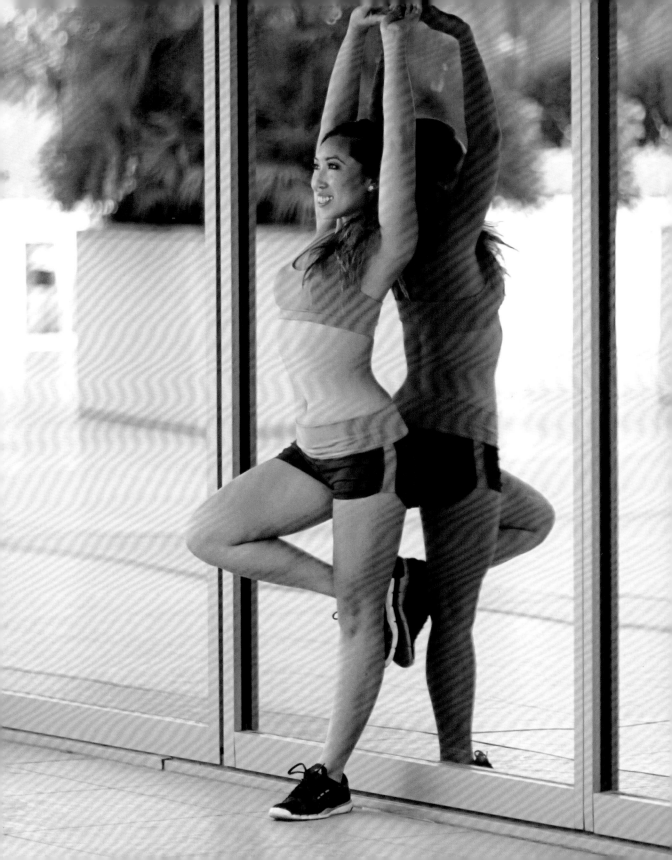

CONTENTS

hey, guys!

I just got back from my Boston Meetup after leading a POP Pilates class of more than 500 crazy enthusiastic POPsters! Mats lined up side by side, people laughing and sweating together for the first time—somehow it feels like we've known one another for years. How does this happen? This is the magic of Blogilates. The magic that you've helped to create. I am overcome with emotion on this plane ride back to L.A., as I massage my cheeks from smiling too much. There are now Sharpie stains all over the fingers on my right hand from signing yoga mats for more than four hours.

I never thought that when I uploaded a simple, unedited Pilates video to YouTube back in 2009 after college graduation that it would lead to any of this. Nor did I intend for it to. But I guess when you follow your passion and decide to live life for happiness—for yourself, for those you love who love you too, and not for the pleasure of others—things just start to flow in your favor.

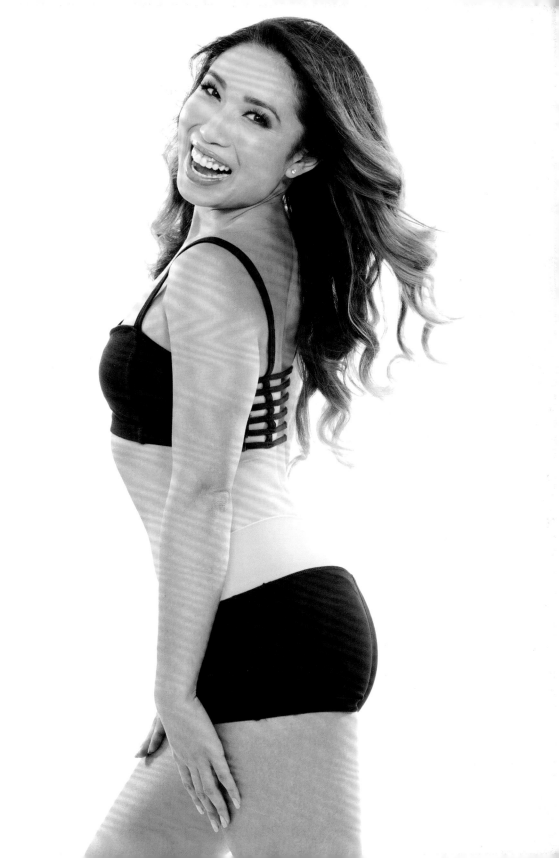

Growing up, I was a superobedient, overachieving child who took home perfect report cards. I was the girl you'd ask to see her homework. As I got older, being that person eventually became very stressful for me, with all the AP classes I was taking along with being captain of the varsity tennis team—but of course, this all made my parents very proud. As a first-generation Vietnamese-Chinese American, I knew that excelling in academics—and life in general—was a big part of our culture. So when it came time to pick a major for college, I was allowed to choose between becoming a doctor or a lawyer. Everything else was unacceptable.

Inside, though, I always wanted to be a fashion designer. I had a natural talent for drawing fashion figures and clothing. At the age of 10, I already had compiled a few 10-inch-thick binders of haute couture, red carpet dresses. When I told my dad I really wanted to go to fashion school, he scolded me so badly. He told me I'd never make money, I'd never be successful, and I would never have any friends. I remember crying forever, until my eyes puffed up so much that I couldn't see. I looked like a sick turtle.

So I took my full-ride scholarship to Whittier College and majored in biology. It wasn't bad, but my heart was missing. My soul felt empty. I thought, "Just get through this, Cassey."

This is when Pilates really became the rock in my life. Between classes and on weekends, I would work out to de-stress myself. Side note: Pilates was something I picked up when I was 16 and had signed myself up for a pageant!

I wanted to tone up quickly, so I started doing Mari Winsor Pilates DVDs from the infomercials and became hooked. Not only did I strengthen my core like mad, I also ended up taking home the crown as Miss Teen Chinatown 2003!

So by the time I was in college, I was a super Pilates enthusiast and was even encouraging my friends to do small sessions with me in the dorm lounge! One day, I was browsing the local classifieds, and I saw an ad for "Pilates Instructor" for a small gym down the street. I knew I probably wasn't qualified, but I was confident and saw no risk in auditioning.

To my surprise, the studio liked my style and offered to pay for my Pilates certification. It was this rare opportunity that sparked everything. They took a chance on a young girl who they believed in.

From that point, I fell head over heels in love with teaching. I'd walk in exhausted from chemistry experiments and lab disasters, lead a class, and leave feeling like a reenergized human being. Pilates did that for me. And it still does. So I will never ever stop teaching. Pilates is and forever will be my rock.

When my father found out I was teaching on the side, he kept telling me to stop and make more time for studying. He said it wouldn't help me in life. So instead, I taught more. And in junior year of college, I dropped out of the only class I still needed to take the MCATs for medical school—organic chemistry. It was a way of sabotaging, or I guess you could say *saving* myself from entering a life I did not want. Now, I won't lie to you and tell you I was strong and stood by that decision. I actually ended up dropping out three times because I was so unsure of myself. It was scary. My parents went berserk.

So I dove deeper into my love affair for design. As a senior in college, I fused my passions for fitness and fashion and I designed a high-end line of yoga bags that I named oGorgeous.

And then my parents stopped talking to me.

Alone and unsure, after graduation I moved to the East Coast to get as far away as I could. I decided to pursue my dreams of becoming part of the fashion world as a buyer. But before I hopped on that one-way plane, I made a farewell workout video for my students in L.A. I hated leaving them, and they hated the thought of missing me, so I thought a good-bye total-body Pilates video would suffice. I filmed the 10-minute Total Body Workout video on a little digital camera and I uploaded it to this site called YouTube.

When I started my corporate job, I became immediately intoxicated with negative energy from my nasty, self-serving fashionista coworkers. Every day my soul was breaking apart. I wasn't meant to be there, and I started losing my biggest asset, my confidence. The only thing I would look forward to each day was teaching my Pilates classes at the local sports club.

Then halfway through the year, a miracle happened. My sister texted me a picture of a blurry page out of *Shape* magazine that kind of resembled a yoga bag. My heart stopped.

I told my coworkers and my boss that I needed to take an early lunch. They rolled their eyes. I ran out to Target and started flipping through the pages of *Shape*. My hands were sweaty and my body was shaking. Then I saw it. It was my Pleated Pocket Yoga Bag, smack dab in the middle of a national magazine feature on top fitness gear. Was this really happening? I started crying. I melted down onto the white linoleum floor.

You know, looking back, this next decision could have made me homeless, but I knew in my heart everything would be okay. I didn't know where I was going or how I was going to make money, but I knew I couldn't be there any longer. So I quit. I just had to get out.

All I had was hope. So with that, I told myself that all I could do now was give myself the chance to succeed, 110 percent or nothing. So, I bought a ticket to China on Friday and left on Sunday, with the aim of looking for a bag manufacturer. It was crazy. I was crazy. It was time to go big.

When I got back from China, I had a three-month development waiting period. I upped my Pilates classes from two times a week to twelve times a week to pay the rent. It was during this period that I truly honed my skills as a better instructor. I became one with the movement, the music, and my students. POP Pilates was born when I realized that Pilates could be more than a slow series of movements, that it could be a challenging dance on the mat. The students seemed to enjoy the sweat and the soreness, so it stuck!

It was also during this time that I started to make more YouTube videos. That one 10-minute Total Body Workout that I uploaded after college had so many comments posted it encouraged me to make more videos. So I listened. And my number of subscribers grew. I listened even closer, and the Blogilates Community began to spread like wildfire, until my channel became the number one most subscribed female fitness channel on YouTube, with hundreds of millions of viewers. Unreal.

I attribute all my success as an instructor to you, my students. Thank you. Because of your enthusiasm and love for health and fitness, I am able to share my passion with millions. It's a dream that I never knew could come true.

And because of you, I am now able to be a fashion designer, too. And make a living. And I have friends. Things that were supposed to be "impossible."

What I want you to know is this: anything is possible as long as you follow what feels right and you stay away from what feels wrong. That way, you end up wiggling your way through life and finding where you belong. And it takes only one person to direct your life the way you want it to play out. That person is YOU.

I hope my story has inspired you to follow your passion, regardless of how many obstacles lie in your path. Regardless of how many people don't believe in you. You've got to believe in yourself. Confidence is your most valuable asset. Don't lose it.

If you show perseverance and follow through, nobody can hold you back. In fact, after Blogilates became an Internet phenomenon, my parents both came to realize that I was okay. They stopped worrying about my future, my education, and my career. They saw that their daughter was happy and flourishing. In the end, that's all that they were trying to secure. I just had to prove that it could be done the nontraditional way. Now, both Mom and Dad come to all of my Meetups and even dress up for the themed workouts! It's so silly but fun. Thanks to you guys for making Blogilates what it is—because of that, I now have back my relationship with my parents.

So, this book is dedicated to you. Thank you for helping me believe in myself and helping me turn Blogilates into the most vibrant and positive fitness community that exists.

I traveled to the gleaming Salt Flats of Utah, to the sun-kissed beaches of Malibu, and to the fiery fall foliage of Massachusetts to photograph this visually stunning POP Pilates book. There were so many challenges induced by Mother Nature that almost made the shoots impossible, but it's in the toughest times that you become the most creative. I'll never forget having to basically shoot the POP Pilates exercises atop a floating piece of something from the hardware store as the wind nearly blew me into the water. Let's just say it was entertaining for everyone.

What I love about the changing seasons is that they allow me to prepare myself for fresh beginnings four times a year! It's a chance to refocus and optimize my goals with the natural flow of the environment. With the seasonal changes in fashion and weather come changes in foods and moods. It's important to take advantage of the changes and use them to motivate you.

This book will take you through the celebrations and challenges of each season. Summer is a time when we all get a little more conscious about our bodies. Use the heat as a reason to exercise outside and to motivate you to work hard for a strong body—and of course, to look confident and sexy in a bikini!

Fall calls for sweaters and covering up, as we drift into a post–summer vacation lull. A little depressing? It doesn't have to be! Fall is a chance to find rhythm and routine, and to discover delicious autumn flavors to keep your eat-clean habits solidly established.

In winter, all we want to do is curl up into a ball to stay warm and EAT. But why don't you heat up by sweating it out instead? And, yes, you can still eat and have a social life. I'll show you foods you can bring to those holiday dinner parties that will have your friends thinking they're cheating—except they're cheating clean!

Then there's spring, the ultimate "New Year, New You" season! You don't have to wait 365 days for this one day to start anew, but if you do decide to begin your fitness journey here, there will be lots of support from friends, family—the whole world! If friendly accountability is what drives you, this is the perfect time to pick a workout buddy and hit it hard!

In this book, you will find a breakdown of my best POP Pilates moves and my favorite recipes that have been used to sculpt millions of strong and healthy bodies all over the world. These routines have been designed to get you into your best physical and mental shape in the comfort of your own home—or even when you're traveling. You won't need any equipment! A mat is recommended, but not necessary. So, no excuses. Understand?

I want you to never have a silly reason for not staying active. It's too easy and too much fun to move! I believe that working out should be something you look forward to—it should not be a chore. That way, it becomes part of your lifestyle. Losing weight and finding your best body will no longer be a battle; it will just be the result of living a happy and healthy life. I wrote this book to help you find a passion in exercising, in the hope that you will inspire your friends to live healthfully, too.

Again, here's a big thank-you to you for making this book possible. I am beyond excited for you to dive into these colorful pages and work out with me.

Ready? Let's get started!
♡ Cassey

a short history of pilates

Joseph Pilates, born in 1880 in Germany, had a natural calling to movement and health—his father was a gymnast and his mother was a practitioner of natural healing. Growing up, Joseph suffered from illness and a frail body, and in an effort to understand and heal himself, he studied anatomy and learned Eastern and Western fitness, including yoga, martial arts, bodybuilding, gymnastics, boxing, recreational sports, ancient Greek and Roman forms of exercise, and even the stretching patterns of animals (inspiration is found *everywhere*).

At age thirty-two, he moved to England, where he taught self-defense at police academies and Scotland Yard until Great Britain entered the First World War. As a German citizen, he was incarcerated, and although at first you would think this was an unfortunate turn of events, he actually took the opportunity to teach other internees his method and mat work. In 1918, an influenza pandemic struck, and while millions died, many of those he taught and trained were not afflicted. Most credit their survival to their being in tip-top shape.

Joseph returned to Germany after the war and worked as a hospital orderly, reconstructing mattresses and using the springs as a form of resistance to rehabilitate those unable to get out of bed, another inspiration that would later shape his method as a whole. He then moved to New York City, where he met his future wife, Clara, who also became his business partner. Together, they opened a studio that attracted local dancers and theater performers because the exercise improved their core (and overall) strength, flexibility, and balance while helping speed the healing of their injuries.

Breathing, proper posture, and the correction of various physical ailments were the focus at Joseph's studio. He seldom taught the same routine twice, taking into account different bodies and the importance of switching up a workout to gain full-body wellness. This naturally progressed into the varied style of Pilates.

In his 1945 book, *Return to Life,* Joseph believed that the stresses of modern life (working, sitting in traffic, school, etc.) harmed a person's pursuit of physical and mental well-being and that practicing Pilates would help someone "return to life," reclaiming balance in the body and peace of mind. Joseph and Clara operated their exercise studio for more than forty years. He dedicated his life's work to restoring the health and vitality of others, just as he had done for himself when he was growing up.

What Is POP Pilates?

The fresh, fun, and upbeat fusion of classical Pilates is mixed with intense core-based mat exercises that will quickly tone your muscles, heighten your posture, and leave you sore—but stronger. The side effects include smiling, laughter, and happiness; all of these have been reported.

POP Pilates has been created by a certified Pilates instructor and fitness star—your very own Cassey!

How Do I Use This Book?

To me, having a hot body means feeling my best, looking my best, and being happy from the inside out. So, I designed this book to ensure that you, also, will be motivated from every possible angle. Be sure to use the fitness and food plans in tandem, and let my motivation keep you going.

There's a solid plan in store for each season that addresses the following four elements:

FITNESS: For each season there are five unique POP Pilates routines, each of which serves a different purpose based on the challenges of that season. Each routine comprises a series of moves, combined for maximum results. For example, in summer we kick it off with an intense Bikini Ab Attack (page 96); in winter, we need a quick Pre-Party Tone-Up session (page 223) before heading out to those holiday parties. This gives you a total of twenty carefully crafted routines and more than 120 different moves that are never repeated—all to keep your muscles surprised.

FOOD: I show you what foods you should eat that will really aid your hard work and boost your progress. The foods are always in season, so you know you'll be saving money, eating fresh, and eating locally. You'll find my beautifully photographed eat-clean recipes along with your own slim-down meal plan to follow. And don't worry—the meal plans are as incredibly delicious as they are satisfying! However, there's also room for a YOLO ("You Only Live Once") meal, when you can go crazy and forget about the calories, the restrictions, and just eat for your soul.

MOTIVATION: If you think you can, you will. It is essential that your mind, body, and goals are all in agreement with a common purpose. If there's misalignment, there's potential for emotional distress and failure. But fear not! Like you, I've been through days when I'm up and days when I'm down—so down that I wanted to give up. And it's in these moments that your resilience needs to shine. But sometimes that resilience needs a little encouragement. When you need some Cassey inspiration, just look for the journal entries I've written to you. Then get up and go!

LIFESTYLE TIPS:
Sprinkled throughout the book are little tricks I use to stay happy, healthy, and strong. These precious gems will make your fitness journey an inspirational experience. I call these "A Note from Cassey." Watch out for them!

SLIM-DOWN MEALS:
In every season you will find my Fast-Track Meal Plans, which are *your* meal plans. You blend the essence of each season (and its produce) with my suggested dishes, along with recipes provided in this book to guide you in your journey. Whether your goal is to slim down, stay fit, or feel better throughout each day, you'll love these menus, which blend my recipes and ideas for simple breakfasts, snacks, lunches, and dinners with staple yummies to help you stay on track.

When you follow these plans paired with the workouts, you will naturally lose weight—because along with the exercise, you will eat clean and control your portions, which ultimately will help you look and feel your best, from the inside out. If you're not looking to lose weight, you can use these plans as reminders and inspiration to help you keep your hot body year-round, and you can use my recipes to guide your creativity in the kitchen.

If you stick to the POP Pilates routines on the Workout Calendars and follow my recipes,

Vegetables
beet greens
bell peppers
bok choy
cabbage
carrots
celery
celery root
leeks
lettuce
mushrooms
onions
parsnips
shallots
spinach
turnips

Fruits
apples
avocados
bananas
lemons
papaya

you will start to see changes in both your body and your mood—within the week. Paired with your own passionate motivation and your desire to sculpt a new healthy lifestyle, success is 100 percent yours. Trust me. If you want it bad enough, you will figure out a way to make it happen.

For each season, I give you a grocery list of what is fresh and in season so you can make the best of the changing months. **ADDITIONALLY, ABOVE IS A LIST OF FRUITS AND VEGGIES FOUND YEAR-ROUND.** Use these anytime, any month, and in any dish you please!

How Do I Pair the Workouts?

BEGINNERS: I want you to work out at least three times a week. Here's your Workout Calendar:

MONDAY	TUESDAY	WEDNESDAY	THURSDAY	FRIDAY	SATURDAY	SUNDAY
1 abs/core workout + 1 legs workout	Rest	1 arms workout + 1 back workout	Rest	1 total body workout + 1 workout of your choice	Cardio for at least 20 minutes. Running, elliptical, cardio dance—anything that gets your heart pumping!	Rest

Of course, you can pick any four days that work with your schedule, but make sure you target these areas!

INTERMEDIATE TO ADVANCED POP PILATES ENTHUSIASTS, OR THOSE OF YOU LOOKING TO LEAN DOWN QUICK:

I want you to strive to work out at least five times a week. Here's your Workout Calendar:

MONDAY	TUESDAY	WEDNESDAY	THURSDAY	FRIDAY	SATURDAY	SUNDAY
4 abs/core workouts of your choice + 20 minutes of cardio	4 legs workouts of your choice + 1 Slim-Down workout	4 arms and back workouts + 20 minutes of cardio	4 abs/core workouts + 1 Slim-Down workout	Any medley of 5 workouts + 10 minutes of cardio	Cardio for at least 1 hour. Running, elliptical, cardio dance—anything that gets your heart pumping!	Rest

Also, if you're looking for more ways to challenge your body, and to avoid plateauing after you've finished the Workout Calendar, print out my monthly workout calendars on www.Blogilates.com. The ones on my blog are paired with my free full-length workout videos, which can all be found on YouTube.com/Blogilates or in the Blogilates Official App in the iTunes and Google Play stores.

What Equipment Do I Need?

All of my bodyweight exercises are meant to challenge you and make you sore without lifting a single dumbbell. A yoga mat is recommended, though, to provide grip and prevent slipping. If you have sensitive joints, you may want to grab a small towel that can be rolled up to serve as cushioning as you perform the moves.

Hot Body on a Budget?

Yes! No one ever said you had to spend hundreds of dollars every month on a fancy gym membership and a cupboard full of supplements. I've heard people complain about how costly it is to live a healthy lifestyle, and you know what? It's simply not true! You can actually save money by eating clean and exercising in the comfort of your own home. I believe that every person can afford to pay attention to his or her well-being.

YOUR HEALTH IS YOUR WEALTH, AFTER ALL.

You can nourish your body with in-season produce, which not only means you're eating local and fresh but also that the things you're buying are on sale. For foods that aren't in season, frozen is another great money-saving option that's just as healthy. Many fruits and vegetables are processed for freezing at their peak ripeness, so they remain nutrient-packed. Try to avoid the canned vegetables, though. These usually have too much sodium, sugar, and other preservatives that degrade their nutrient quality. If you are using canned beans, make sure you are purchasing low sodium versions and rinsing thoroughly before use.

For exercise, you don't really need cardio machines and big, shiny equipment to get fit. Before humans had cars to travel in and computers to be glued to, we were naturally more active. Just walking can actually help you lose weight or maintain a healthy body. Parking your car farther away from the entrance of the mall or taking the stairs instead of the elevator are simple ways you can sneak exercise into your daily routine.

But it doesn't stop there. There are endless at-home exercises you can perform to truly sculpt your best body. POP Pilates does not require anything but a yoga mat to cushion your body against the floor. All of the exercises utilize your own body as a weight to help slim

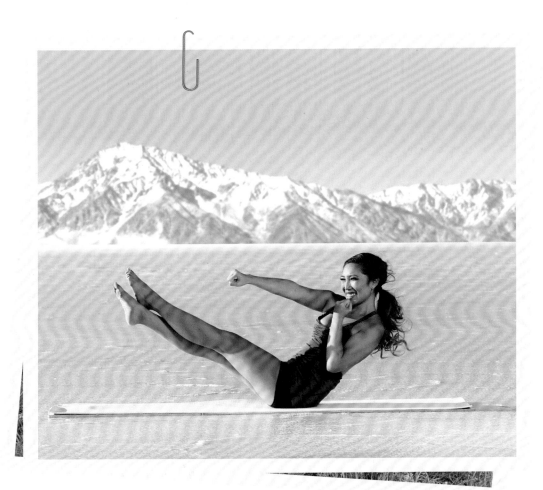

your waist, firm up your abs, lift your booty, tone your arms, and sculpt your legs. You will be sore from my exercises because I'm going to show you how to use your muscles in a way they've never been used before. But this is what's going to change your body and transform your physique.

Common POP Pilates Vocabulary

This is a preview of a few key terms you'll find I use over and over in this book. They are critical components of the hot body exercises!

PILATES STANCE

This is a common starting position we use to engage your upper abs during many of the exercises. Beginning with your back on the mat, lift your shoulders and head off the ground, arms by your hips, reaching for your thighs. Your head should be lifted enough so that your eyes are staring in front of you, not at the ceiling. Your lower back should be pressed into the mat. It is important to get this technique correct or else you could end up feeling tension in your neck.

PILATES C-CURVE

When performing moves where we roll our spine down to the mat from a sitting position, we must be conscious of our lower back. Imagine that you are sitting tall, then someone hugs your belly and pulls you back while you're reaching forward. This helps you further engage your abs in an effective manner.

TABLETOP

This is another common placement of the legs in which the knees are stacked over the hips at a 90-degree angle with the shins parallel to the floor, toes pointed.

PLANK

This is an amazing core-strengthening exercise in which you are balanced on your hands and your toes (or a combination of the former, with elbows and knees for beginners). Your body should look like the wooden plank that pirates used to make their victims walk—firm with tailbone and pelvis tucked in. There should be no dip in the lower back and the butt should be in line with the back and the legs.

SIDE PLANK

This is a beautiful and strong exercise for your shoulders and obliques since you balance your body on a single palm and single foot. Beginners may start on their knee to build strength.

CHILD'S POSE

This is a relaxed position in which your chest is resting on your thighs, knees bent underneath you, head resting on the mat, and arms stretched forward.

PLIÉ

A classic ballet move in which your feet are turned outward, as you bend your knees into a squat, while keeping your back straight. This move is great for toning your thighs and glutes.

CORE

I will say "core" a lot in this book, and you've surely heard it a million times in my workout videos. This refers to your abs, your obliques, and your low abs. Basically, imagine tying a string around your waist. Anything that touches that string is a part of your core. In Pilates, the core is a big focus, as it is the center of your balance and where all of your strength emanates from.

PART 1
THE

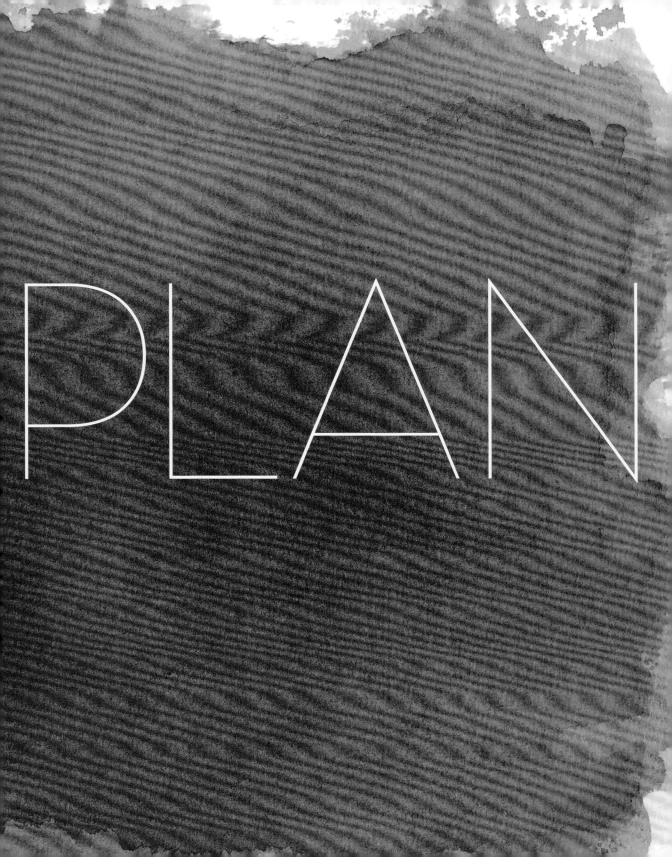

PLAN

how to eat for a hot body, year-round

EATING CLEAN 101

Before we get into the moves, let's talk about how to fuel your body. These tips will have you feeling energized, strong, and powerful.

Our bodies react to food, and the way we eat is reflected through the health of our skin, hair, and nails, as well as internally; that health also shows up in our energy level, our weight, and our overall longevity.

Eating clean is creating your meals the way people did before machines mass-processed all of it. It's walking into a grocery store and putting yourself back in touch with nature by purchasing fresh produce, grass-fed meats, whole grains, and unsweetened beverages.

That's a key part of having a hot body year-round. I provide you with the tools to achieve a year (actually, could be a lifetime) of clean eating by learning how to shop and pick the freshest produce that's in season to create easy and yummilicious meals! Let's begin with navigating your supermarket.

Grocery chains place clean, natural, and perishable items on the perimeters of the store, and these include produce, dairy, and butcher items. Commercially packaged items are in the middle aisles, placed on shelves and packed with preservatives, which allow them to sit on those shelves for a long time and not go bad. These processed foods are filled with sodium, saturated fats, and chemical preservatives. They are also bogged down with additives and dyes that mimic natural flavors but will not fade over time. The more bogged down these foods are with "ingredients" (check the labels!), the more bogged down your body will feel.

Help your body sustain a balanced, clean feel by incorporating natural and whole foods into your diet. Here are my tips for clean shopping!

✳ Shop the perimeter for your fresh items, including produce, dairy, meats, tofu, and so on.

✳ Be mindful of the ingredient list on the packaged items you buy. If the ingredient list is longer than your grocery list, it's probably not healthy. Also, if you don't recognize some of the words on the list, most likely they're not natural ingredients. For example:

- Let's say you're buying oatmeal, and the ingredients include flavorings aside from "oats"; pick up another box. You'll learn how to flavor your oatmeal later on, in tasty recipes such as Sweet Potato Oatmeal (page 184), with vanilla, cinnamon, and maple syrup.

✳ Eat lean, grass-fed meats or wild-caught fish that aren't bulked up with hormones, nitrites, and additives. Our meat and fish factories are overcrowded and a lot of the time the inhabitants are feeding off of each other's waste and grime, which means we are eventually eating dirty food. To avoid this, pay attention to what you are buying and look for quality food, even if it costs a little more. For example:

- For meats, look for labels that say "cage free," "grass fed," "no nitrites added," or "hormone free."
- For fish, look for labels that indicate "wild caught" or "line caught."

✳ Incorporate whole grains into your diet, including steel-cut oats, quinoa, farro, or brown rice.

- Try to avoid "instant" items when you can. The more "instant" it is, the more it's been processed and stripped of its nutrients or fiber.

✳ Look at the added sugars and then reconsider.

- Whole-grain cereals and granolas should have less than 8 grams of sugar. If you want it sweeter, take it home and spruce it up, like in my Lemon-Cherry Quinoatmeal (page 82). I add sweetness by incorporating fruit and cinnamon.

Now that you have filled your grocery bags with wholesome goodies, you're prepped for dynamic breakfasts, lunches, dinners, and even desserts to cater to your sweet cravings. It's really important to have a blast in the kitchen, experimenting with flavors and seasonal harvests. You'll see in my recipes, like the Flourless Pizza with Figs and Rosemary (page 135), that when there is a shift in the season, you can swap the figs and rosemary for squash and sage (winter) or blackberries (spring). For lunch in the fall, you'll be prepped with my Turkey Quesadilla (page 186) that's served with cranberry salsa. Well, guess what? Come summer you can swap those tart little cranberries for tomatoes.

Here are some of my favorite tips for the kitchen that will slim down your meals and drinks without compromising flavor:

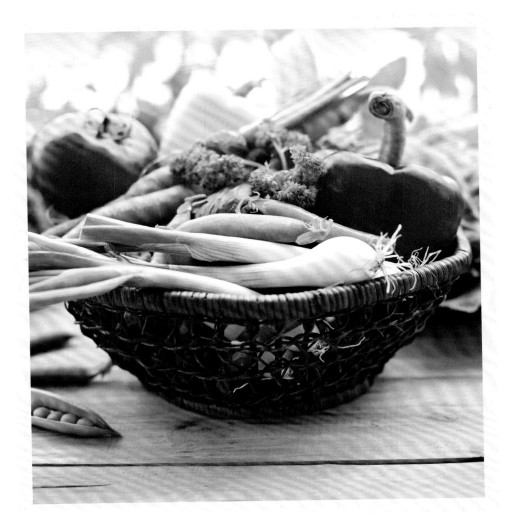

* Replace salt and flavor your foods with herbs such as parsley, rosemary, sage, basil, mint, dill, chives, cilantro, marjoram, and more! Learn what herbs pair best—that is, parsley and basil, or mint and oregano, and have at it!

* Nix the sodas and flavor your own waters by adding lemon, lime, orange, ginger, cucumber, strawberries, and so on.

* Skip the animal fats, like butter, cheese, heavy creams, and whole milk, and find alternatives, like coconut oil, olive oil, nuts, and avocado.

* Experiment with exotic veggies and fruits! Rummage through your pantry and find things you can make with those new, natural foods! Have fun! Eat the rainbow (not Skittles) and find your health's pot of gold.

Cassey's Daily Meal Plan

Here's a sneak peek at how I fill my plate in the course of a day. These are a few of my go-to recipes—and there will be many more coming, in each season's chapter.

BREAKFAST:
Metabolic Supercharge Smoothie

INGREDIENTS

1 cup chopped kale

1 frozen sliced banana

1 cup crushed ice

Juice of 1 lemon

½ cup 2% plain Greek yogurt

½ cup unsweetened almond milk

¼ teaspoon cayenne pepper

DIRECTIONS

Place all the ingredients in a blender and spin until smooth. Pour into a tall glass and serve.

MAKES 1

SNACK:

Small handful of baby carrots • 2 tablespoons organic unsweetened peanut butter

LUNCH:
Fresh Tacos

INGREDIENTS

- 4 ounces 99% fat-free ground turkey
- ½ bell pepper, seeded and chopped
- ½ onion, chopped
- 5 leaves of iceberg lettuce
- 1 lime, cut in half
- Pico de gallo or salsa

DIRECTIONS

Place the turkey, bell pepper, and onion in a small nonstick skillet and sauté for 5 minutes, until cooked through. Shape your lettuce leaves into "taco shells" and fill with the meat mixture. Squeeze a little lime juice on top and spoon on some pico de gallo or salsa.

MAKES 5

SNACK:

½ cup nonfat plain Greek yogurt • 2 strawberries, hulled and sliced • 1 tablespoon raw sunflower seeds

---

DINNER:
Salmon Bowl

INGREDIENTS

- ½ cup cooked quinoa or brown rice
- 2 cups steamed green beans or asparagus spears
- 1 (4-ounce) baked salmon fillet
- Sriracha hot sauce (optional)

DIRECTIONS

In a bowl, layer the quinoa or rice with vegetables and salmon. Top with the Sriracha, if desired.

SERVES 1

FOODS FOR BEAUTIFUL HAIR, SKIN, AND NAILS

You can create beauty from the inside out by honing in on what you are consuming, which is why clean eating is so important. Certain foods have nutritious properties that not only boost your health and energy but also promote strong nails, luxurious hair, and clear, soft, and young-looking skin.

The foods you eat are the best resource for toning your skin. Our bodies depend on nutrient-rich foods to thrive, glow, and fight the outward signs of disease and aging. Eating nutritious foods will help your skin fight acne, reduce redness and inflammation, aid in moisture issues, and even slow down the signs of aging. Your skin, nails, and hair are all part of the integumentary organ system, which protects the body from damage such as loss of water or abrasion, so it is important to feed this system to enhance their look and function.

The following is a list of hair-boosting, nail-enriching, skin-glowing nutrients and foods to add to your grocery lists and cooking habits in order to help boost your beauty:

Vitamin A/beta carotene Helps to turn over dead skin cells by encouraging new ones, while also strengthening the nails. It also prevents dandruff, dry skin, and flaking.

* Found in apricots, asparagus, broccoli, cantaloupe, carrots, eggs, raw endive, kale, leaf lettuce, liver, milk, mustard greens, pumpkin, spinach, squash, sweet potatoes, tomatoes, watermelon.

Vitamin B A family of eight vitamins; they protect your skin from environmental damage and enhance your nail growth.

* Found in beef, blue cheese, clams, dairy, eggs, fish, milk. (Note: vitamin B is not typically found in plant foods.)

Vitamin C For youthful skin, healthy hair, and strong nails.

* Found in blueberries, kiwis, lemons, grapefruit, oranges, tomatoes, strawberries, peppers, pomegranate, broccoli, Brussels sprouts.

Vitamin D Aids in strengthening the hair and nails.

* Found in fish oils, tuna, salmon, and is absorbed from sunlight.

Vitamin E Protects your skin from ultraviolet light and free-radical damage.

* Found in almonds, asparagus, avocados, brazil nuts, broccoli, corn, hazelnuts, nut oils, seeds, wheat germ.

Calcium Strengthens nails and promotes hair growth and reproduction.

* Found in almonds, Brazil nuts, broccoli, caviar, cheese, cottage cheese, kelp, milk, salmon, turnip greens, yogurt.

Omega-3 fatty acids Help your skin look younger and healthier, and also keep your scalp hydrated.

 ✳ Found in salmon, walnuts, avocados, cauliflower.

Antioxidants Aid in hair growth and preventing hair loss, reverse skin discoloration, and protect the skin from the sun.

 ✳ Found in green tea, dark chocolate, black coffee, berries.

Zinc and iron Prevent hair loss and keep the skin and scalp from flaking, while giving nails the protein and iron they need.

 ✳ Found in eggs, lean meats, yogurt, legumes.

WHY DO WOMEN LOVE SWEETS?

Let's face it—women are sugar fiends. I know some women who must eat something sweet after every meal or they cannot focus. It doesn't help that we are all tempted by sugary items everywhere we look—froyo, candy, sodas, chocolate, chocolate, and back to froyo, sometimes all in one day!

Traditional Chinese medicine explains the sugar craving as an imbalanced Spleen Qi. Qi is the energy force that allows the organs to work seamlessly together, and the spleen is responsible for digestion, metabolism, and energy production (among many other things). When people are spleen deficient, they crave sweet flavors; it's just like when someone's liver is imbalanced, he or she craves the sour taste.

Women tend to be more spleen deficient than men because the energy of the spleen is used to make blood. Because a woman's monthly cycle depends on the spleen, we crave sugar more often.

To retrain your palate to ward off these sweet cravings, you can, slowly but surely, replace artificial sweeteners (Splenda, Sweet 'n Low, Equal) and refined sugars (white sugar, sugar in the raw, brown sugar) with naturally sweet items like fruits, agave, grade B maple syrup, and molasses. Then you can cut back on your intake of sweets as a whole. For example, you can replace candy toppings during your froyo trips with fresh fruit, then also cut back on the frequency of your trips. (Instead of going seven days a week, go once.) Make it your YOLO meal.

In truth, your body doesn't *need* candy, so don't let your cravings fool you. Focus on what your body needs and create ways to fool your cravings!

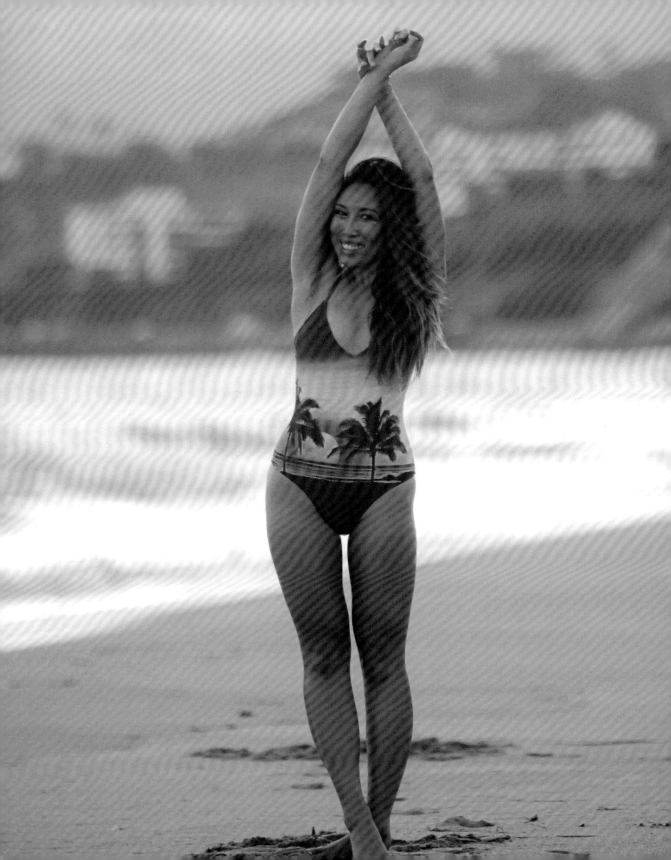

How Much Water Should I Drink?

Why is water so important? First, water is our life source; it fuels our internal organs, allowing them to function with vitality and spirit. Water makes up 60 percent of our body weight. It flushes toxins out of our vital organs, carries nutrients to our cells, and provides a moist environment for the tissues in our ears, nose, and throat.

Throughout the day, our bodies lose water in different ways, including sweating and even breathing. It is important, therefore, to replace that water to keep the body fully hydrated.

WATERLATES RULES

- Drink 9 (8-ounce) cups a day.
  - » Since you will be exercising, add a cup or two to replenish the sweat you lose.
  - » Drink 1 cup of water at the beginning and 1 cup at the end of each day.
  - » In the morning, your body wakes up after 8 hours (if you're sleeping enough) without water entering its system. Your body needs that water ASAP! Revitalize those organs—awaken them and freshen them with a tall glass.
  - » In the evening, prepare yourself for slumber with the 1-cup nightcap.
- Keep a large quart bottle of water (32 ounces/4 cups) with you throughout the day so you can easily track how much you are drinking. (That means you need to fill the bottle twice!)
- Flavor your water: add natural flavorings to enhance the water-drinking experience. Try sliced cucumber, lemon, ginger, lime, fresh strawberries.
  - » Replace your sodas NOW!
  - » Lemon detoxifies, flushes out your system, aids in digestion! Because of its vitamin C and antioxidant properties, it even helps clear your skin, so freely add it to your H_2O.

Drink your 2 quarts of water daily and your internal organs, skin, hair, nails, and energy levels will live happily ever after.

how to stay motivated while you build your hot body

FITNESS IS A JOURNEY

Fitness is not an overnight endeavor or a quick success. Fitness is time, patience, humility, effort, motivation, commitment, perseverance, support—the list is as long as a marathon, but just like any journey, you lace up your shoes, review your goal, and GO!

During your fitness journey, open your heart to the lessons that will present themselves to you and, more important, expand your ability to learn from them. For instance, on day one, it might be difficult for you to do a Pistol Squat without modifications. Don't worry and don't get discouraged! With a good attitude you will conquer those squats over time and with practice.

Living a fit and healthy life is a thoughtful process, and getting into the groove of it can often be tough. It's about transforming bad habits into good habits and training your body to become stronger, healthier, and more energetic. Soon, it will all come together as a natural part of your everyday life, but it takes thought, effort—and it *does* take time. You can't just think you're going to wake up and be a changed person; that goes for any aspect of life. But this is especially the case for fitness!

Although there is no "end" to your fitness journey, you will find that your positive and healthy decisions will seamlessly become part of your everyday routine. Your body will be stronger and so will your mind. It's the story, the challenges, and the successes that bring you to where you want to be and to who you want to become. Embrace the hurt, inhale the lessons, and train insane or remain the same!

HOW TO MAKE YOUR DREAMS COME TRUE

A lot of people want to achieve their dreams and be "successful." But do you know what separates a successful individual from the rest of us? It's saying you want to do something—and actually DOING IT. Sure, it may be scary, but if you believe in yourself, there is actually very little risk.

Why is this? Because your confidence is your best asset. And if you're not going to believe in yourself, who will?

If you fail, you learn. That is, you learn to do it right the next time. When you succeed, no one is going to remember how many times you failed before you got there. The only thing that matters is that you got there.

Here are my rules for making sure your dreams become a reality:

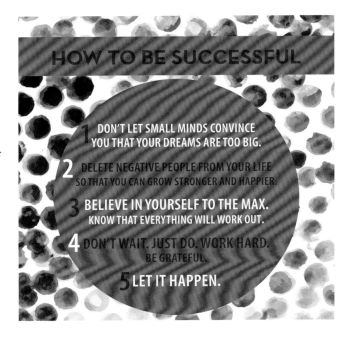

* Don't let small minds convince you that your dreams are too big.
* Delete negative people from your life so that you can grow stronger and happier.
* Believe in yourself to the max. Know that everything will work out.
* Don't wait. Just do. Work hard. Be grateful.
* Let it happen.

GOAL SETTING

A goal is a guide as well as a destination. It helps you stay on track and leads you to the destination of your choosing. This may be to learn and achieve new things, to discover a new strength, to strengthen a weakness, to shape up, to drink more water, to try a new ingredient—whatever that goal is, make sure that you are always evolving toward it.

Here are my tips for making any dream turn into a reality:

* Pick a goal that you can actually achieve—something that excites you and something that is tangible: I want to rule the world versus I want to rule these jeans!
* Write the goal down and tack it in a visible place so that every morning it says "Hello! It's me! Your goal. Good luck today!"

* Tell your friends and family about this goal so that they can encourage you, motivate you, and cheer you on.
* Set a deadline for reaching your goal!
* Map out the goal as a series of mini goals or small steps. When you achieve one step, you move to the next step. For example, "I want to slim down for those jeans!"

    Step 1: Swap soda for lemon/lime water.

    Step 2: Follow *Hot Body Year-Round*.

    Step 3: Eat clean!

    Step 4: Pick your dream jeans.

    Step 5: Set your next goal.

* If you reach a bump in the road, take a deep breath and find a way to continue toward it. Don't get discouraged. Use your support (you know, those friends and family you told) to bring you positive energy and help!
* Avoid putting pressure on yourself. Goals are not meant to stress you out, so the moment you feel stressed, reevaluate your progress and try mapping out the goal again.

YOUR POTENTIAL IS LIMITLESS!

Weight Loss vs. Muscle Building

We all have different goals as we explore our fitness journeys. For many women, the goal is to lose weight. However, please understand that the number on your scale is not everything.

I encourage you to focus on building muscle as you shed fat. "Won't I get bulky?" you ask. Nope! You won't. Women are not engineered to gain muscle mass like men do, and even if we were, we'd need to eat so much protein and lift weights like maniacs.

The reason why you want to build lean muscle is because it actually speeds up your metabolism, helping you burn more calories throughout the day even at rest. Any weight-bearing exercises, like the ones you see in our POP Pilates routines, will help you build muscle.

Remember to also eat clean, as that will contribute to 80 percent of your physique. This is what will help you lean out so that your definition will show more prominently.

Lastly, remember to have fun! The more you enjoy your exercises and the food you make, the less you will stress about your body and the more responsive it will be to these lifestyle changes.

building your
hot body

POP PILATES BEST PRACTICE

Before I go into the more technical aspects of the POP Pilates practice, remember that I just want you to bring your *best self* to the mat. As long as you try to follow through on every exercise with passion and purpose, you will be doing POP Pilates as I have always envisioned it.

What distinguishes POP Pilates from traditional Pilates is how much fun you'll have during the workouts and how happy you'll feel after them. You will be infectiously empowered and glowing with positive energy, able to do whatever it is you want to achieve! It's just something magical that happens when you move your body like this.

FIVE POP PILATES BEST PRACTICES

1. Abs always tight! Allow all energy to emanate from there. Pull your belly button into your spine, drawing your abs in and up. Imagine that you're wearing a corset.

2. Be graceful like a dancer! Shoulders away from the ears as you lengthen and relax your neck. Energy should come from the core and release through the tips of your fingers and your tippy toes. Imagine lengthening, reaching, and extending your body toward leanness.

3. Breathe! Exhale when you're on the difficult part of the move and inhale as you go back to the resting or starting position.

4. Be aware! Create a purposeful connection between your mind and your body by concentrating on the muscle being worked and why you want it to perform for you.

This will not only help you learn how to control your body, but it will also help you enjoy the details of the practice more.

5. Believe in yourself! Know that you are stronger than you think and that you can push yourself to do anything you want. Just tell yourself you can, and you will.

If you're new to Pilates, you may find that your neck will feel heavy from the motion of lifting your abs into Pilates Stance. Over time, as you strengthen your core, this will no longer be a problem, but in the beginning I suggest you place a couple towels, a small pillow, or a yoga block right behind your head to relieve the weight of your head pulling down.

Another trouble spot may be your lower back. This area tends to create an uncomfortable hollowed arch during lower body exercises like the Double-Leg Lift (page 49). Again, this is a result of an untrained core. So, to provide support until you get stronger, you may either place both your hands underneath your tailbone or place a rolled towel right in the arch of your lower back.

That's all you will need for POP Pilates! The goal is to use your body as your weight and define your muscles, better your posture, and increase your flexibility with moves you can do anywhere, without a gym.

You're going to be amazing!

I know it.

THE IMPORTANCE OF A STRONG CORE

Our core is our center. It is the structural pillar for how we move, connecting our upper and lower body. A ballerina's poise depends on her core, but so does your getting out of bed! Having that sturdy structure for everyday tasks and fitness is crucial. Strengthening the core and learning how to use it to your advantage will improve overall balance, stability, and posture so much so that, when you walk into a room, everyone will unconsciously straighten up to emulate you.

How do you use your core? You use it every day, as you pick up your workout clothes from the floor; do the dishes; or balance in high heels and then bend over to take them off after a long night! These are some tasks that summon your core:

ON A DATE When you feel those butterflies fluttering about in your stomach, transfer them to the core as the positive/strong energy to present yourself in a confident manner; you engage your core to stand tall and straight.

STANDING Aside from your legs, your body needs your core to stand upright. Imagine no core—you would keel over at the street corner, waiting to cross.

EXERCISE Building the power in your core will automatically stabilize your body and allow your agility to be at its best. With a well-working core, your form will be stellar, your flexibility will allow you to move easier, and your nimble self will be able to move with proper form, whether it's holding a Single-Legged Bridge Pulse (page 57) or rockin' the Oil Rigger (page 118)!

So, drop down and give me a one-minute Plank and embrace the burn that will guide your body to move seamlessly.

WORKING OUT = HAPPY MIND

You push hard for 30 straight minutes, a puddle of sweat has gathered on the floor beneath you, your legs are shaking like a mild earthquake, and the cute little bun on the top of your head is now slopped to the side, somewhere in the midst of frizzies. It's not your best moment.

Yet, after composing yourself (and your bun), there's a terrific lightness that overcomes your body and mind, and you feel like you're floating—ah! the high of post-exercise.

Exercise, as I'm sure you've noticed, helps reduce stress and brings on happiness. It wards off anxiety, boosts energy, and promotes self-esteem. Some people say an apple a day keeps the doctor away. I'd say the Burpee Kick (page 77) does that, too.

In a physical-psychological study on women, researchers showed that physical activities affect women's behavior and temper, decrease their stress and anxiety, and increase their self-esteem. Well, look at that!

During a workout, your body creates endorphins that shoot up to your brain, knocking down the doors and giving it a big hug. Endorphins act as our body's natural medicine for reducing pain, both physically and mentally. Their chemical makeup is similar to that of opiates, which are drugs that alleviate pain and have the ability to make us feel good. Endorphins, like opiates, are associated with mood changes, and because exercise releases endorphins to the brain, they give that euphoric feeling we know as the "runner's high."

So, tighten up those shoes, my friends, and get those endorphins moving!

PART 2 THE SEAS

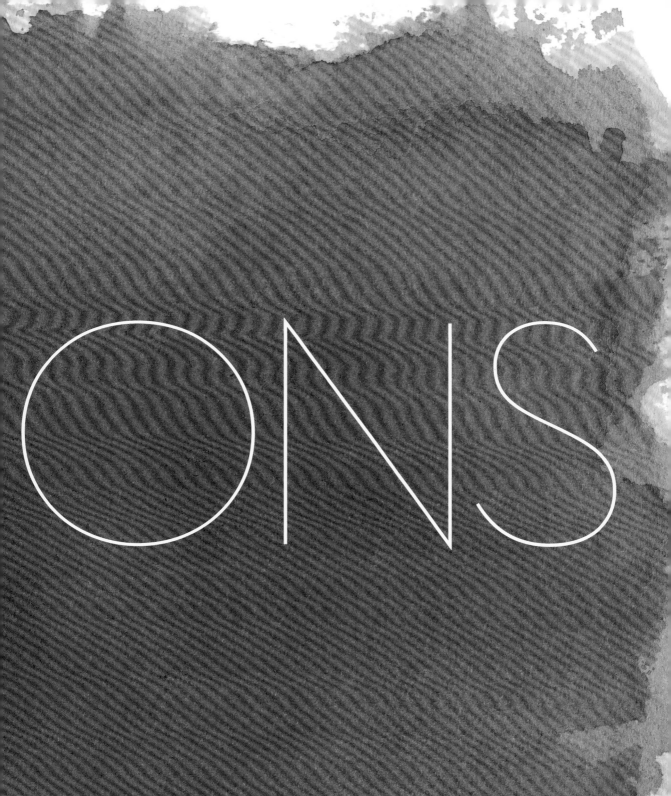

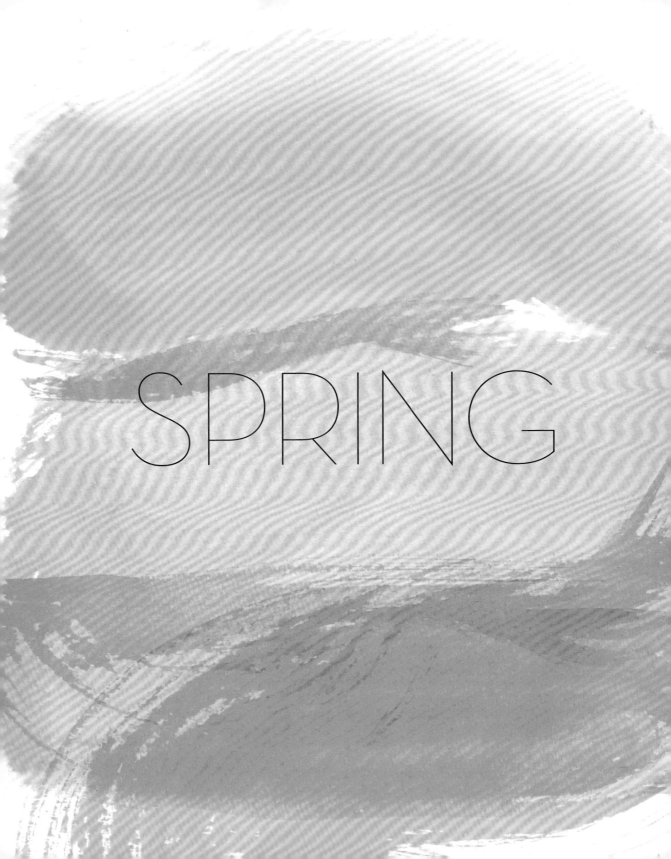

SPRING

Spring
time to bloom, invigorate, start fresh

Ahhhh . . . take in your first fresh breath of air and inhale the purity that comes with every beautiful spring season. The world around you is coming alive, awakening from the slumber of winter. What better time than now to transform your body with the inspiring environment blossoming around you?

With spring comes brilliant color. The dreary clouds have drifted away, the snow has melted, and the sun is warm, signaling the flowers to open and the fruits and veggies to form for a succulent harvest to come. Listen to your body closely this season and hear its natural cravings for those colors and flavors, especially in the foods it needs.

Since the holidays are over, for most of us there aren't as many temptations around, like pies and cakes, so now it's your time to really get back on track. You differentiate your body's calling for a want—like candy or french fries—and instead listen (and learn) what it needs, like the glorious basket of berries that are fresh and on sale!

I believe it's always best to harmonize with nature. It actually makes accomplishing things a lot easier, like going with the flow of a river instead of going against the current! Knowing that, tell me what you've always wanted to achieve. Go ahead, be honest. It can be physical, mental, spiritual, or just plain silly! Got it? Okay, now commit. Promise yourself that this spring you will give yourself what you need to transform your body and mind into the strongest and happiest person it can be.

SPRING MOVES

Spring is simply the perfect time to reinvigorate yourself, just as the earth is doing, so let your muscles play with the warmth of the sun. Buy some fresh-cut flowers to add a bit of nature's simple beauty to your everyday life, so that every morning your first breath will be an inspiring whiff of nature.

WORKOUT #1: RESTORE THE CORE

This workout will engage your core and work your stomach to get your abs in magic shape before you know it. We start with Genie Abs to warm up and engage your muscles. It's going to be a challenge, but your core will thank me later!

GENIE ABS X 15
WORKS: LOWER ABS

A Start with your back and head rested on the mat, arms crossed like a genie and legs twisted in Eagle pose (your knees and ankles should be crossed over). Beginners, you can simply cross your knees until you become more flexible.

B Tighten your ab muscles and lift your knees up to touch your forearms, while keeping your head rested.

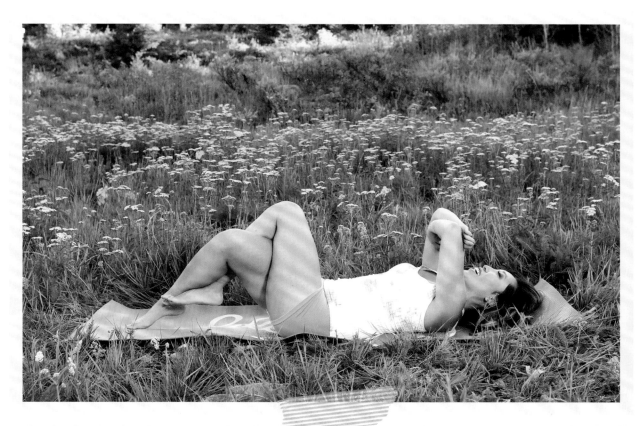

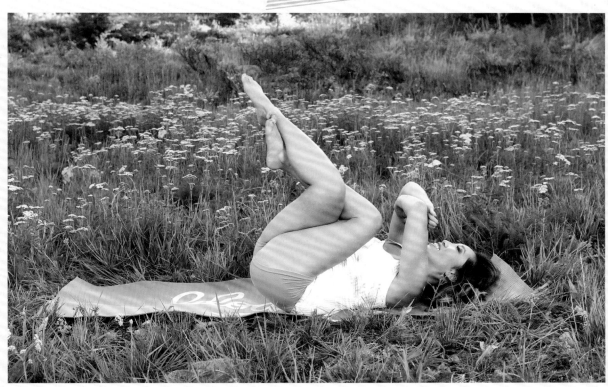

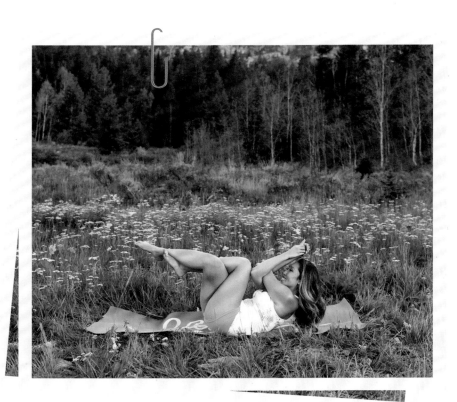

EAGLE CRUNCH X 15
WORKS: ALL ABS

A Begin with your back on the mat, arms in Eagle pose, elbows twisted, and hands clasped. Bring your legs into Eagle pose as well, with knees crossed and ankles twisted.

B Go into a double crunch. Make sure you lift your upper back off the mat and bring your elbows into your knees as your tailbone lifts.

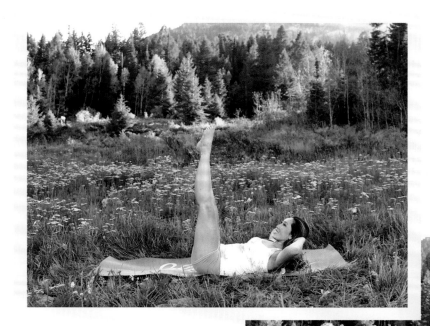

DOUBLE-LEG LIFT X 15
WORKS: LOWER ABS

A Bring your hands behind your head, elbows wide, lower back pressed into the mat, with legs lifted into the air. Keep your legs straight, heels pressed together and your toes pointed to create a V shape. Beginners, you may bend your knees.

B Tighten your abs and press your lower back into the mat as you bring your legs down as far as you can. Then slowly bring them back up toward start.

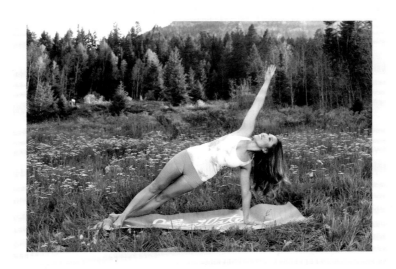

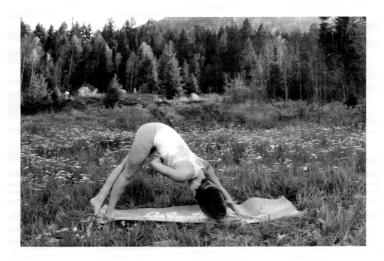

BALLERINA TWIST X 10 EACH SIDE
WORKS: SHOULDERS, OBLIQUES

A Start in a Side Plank, with your bottom arm directly under your shoulder and your upper arm lifted toward the sky, top leg crossed over and in front of the bottom ankle.

B Thread your upper arm underneath your oblique and push your rear toward the sky. Then return to start.

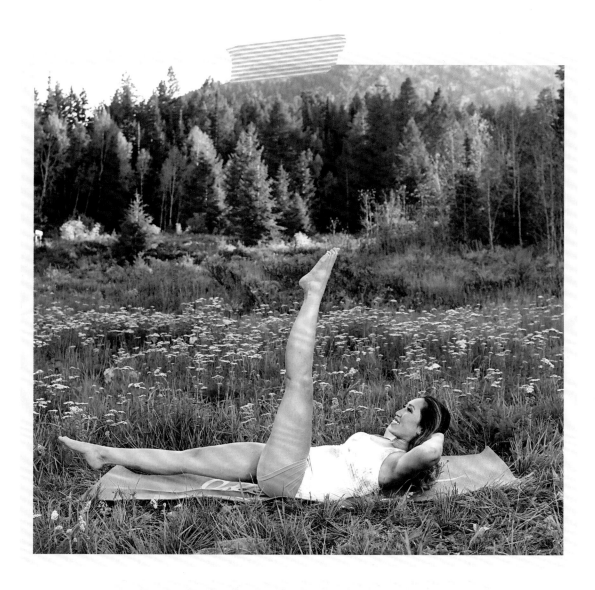

CHEERLEADER L CRUNCH X 10 EACH LEG
WORKS: UPPER ABS, LOWER ABS

A Remain on your back in Pilates Stance, lower back pressed into the mat. Keep your legs straight, toes pointed, one leg out parallel to the floor, other leg up to the sky. Elbows pointed outward, crunch up.

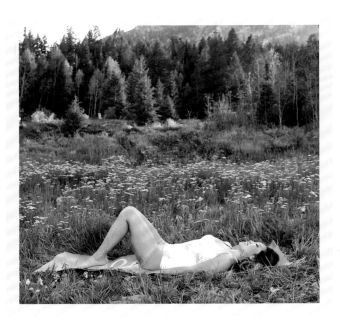

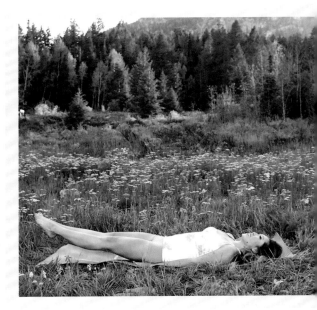

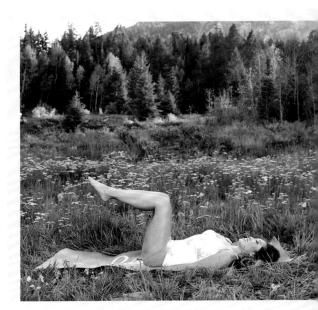

SAND DIGGING X 15
WORKS: LOWER ABS

A Start in Pilates Stance, with your shoulder blades lifted up, eyes looking forward, and lower back pressed into the mat. Your knees will begin in Tabletop position with shins parallel to the floor. Point your toes and drag them on the mat until your legs are straight in front of you, then circle back to return to Tabletop position.

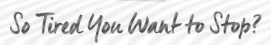

So Tired You Want to Stop?

Keep going! Even for one more rep or 10 more seconds than you think you can last. You are stronger than you think.

WORKOUT #2: DAISY DUKES DERRIERE

You'll be wearing short shorts in no time with this total glute-busting workout. Each move targets your entire upper leg region all the way up to your core, to shape and tighten your butt—so you can feel confident in your Daisy Dukes!

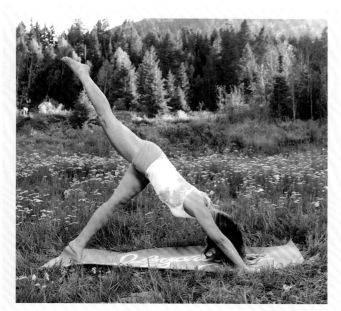

RAINBOW BUTT
X 10 EACH LEG
WORKS: GLUTEUS

A Get into a Down Dog position with hands in front of you, chest pressed toward the mat, heels pressed down. Try to flatten your upper back. Raise your right leg in the air—try not to swivel the hips! Keep them aligned. Beginners, you may start this exercise on all fours. Palms underneath your shoulders, knees hip width apart, back flat.

B Tap your right big toe on the right outside of your mat, then lift it up into the air, draw a rainbow with your leg, and then land that big toe on the left outside of your mat.

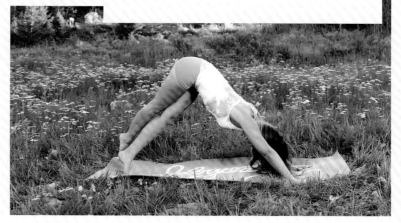

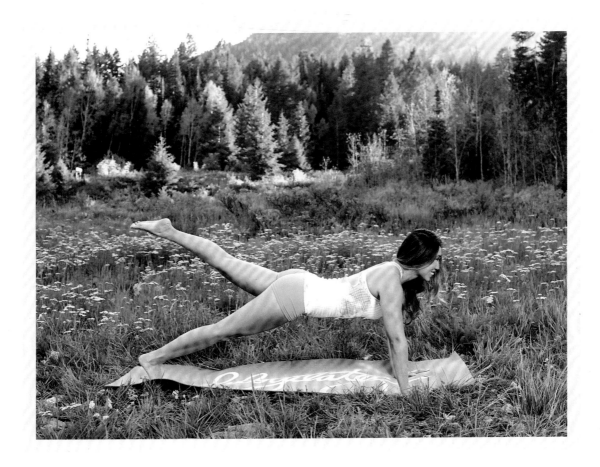

PLANK BUTT PULSE X 12 EACH LEG
WORKS: CORE, GLUTEUS

A Start in Plank on your palms and feet, abs engaged, pelvis tucked. If you are a beginner, go on your elbows and toes. Beginners, you may also start on your knees, palms underneath shoulders, knees hip width apart, back flat.

B Lift your left leg up, squeeze your glutes, raise and pulse your leg up into the air.

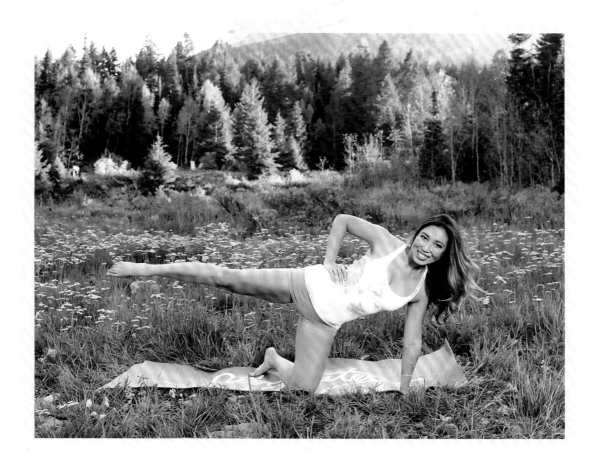

MINI CIRCLE X 20 FORWARD, 20 BACKWARD, EACH LEG
WORKS: INNER THIGHS, OUTER THIGHS, GLUTEUS

A Balance on your side with your left palm and left knee on the mat, pelvis and chest straight forward, right hand on your hip. Beginners, you may lie on your side with one hand underneath your head, one hand in front of you, to balance the body. From here, you can begin the leg circles.

B Lift your right leg up to hip height and begin to circle your whole leg forward. Try not to drop the leg.

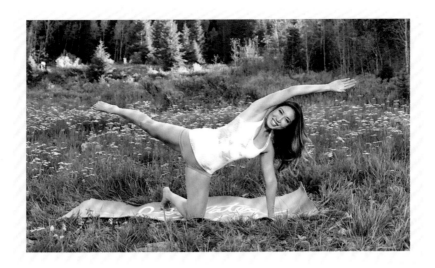

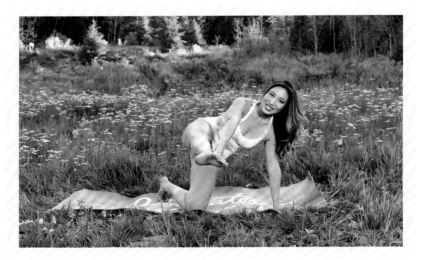

FOLDING TOE TOUCH X 12 EACH SIDE
WORKS: CORE, GLUTEUS

A Balance on your side with your left palm on the mat, left knee on the mat, pelvis and chest straight forward, right arm overhead, and right leg lifted hip height.

B Bring your right leg in front of you and touch your right toes with your right hand. This should be a crunching motion with extended limbs. To make this more advanced and to target the gluteus more, place your right hand behind your head and just perform the leg motion.

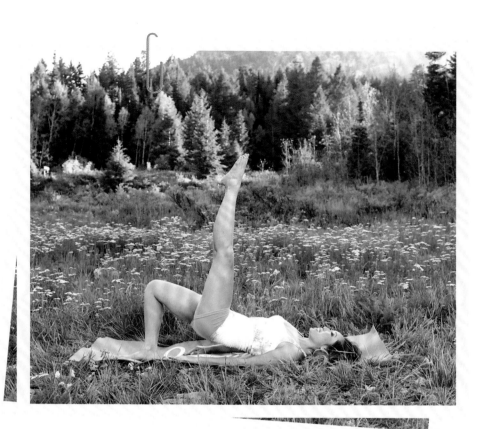

SINGLE-LEGGED BRIDGE
PULSE X 15 EACH LEG
WORKS: GLUTEUS

A Begin in Bridge with your upper back on the mat, hands relaxed and outstretched toward your hips, pelvis and glutes up in the air, knees bent, feet flat.

B Lift your left leg into the air, perpendicular to the mat, toes pointed. Lift your glutes up, keeping that lifted leg in place.

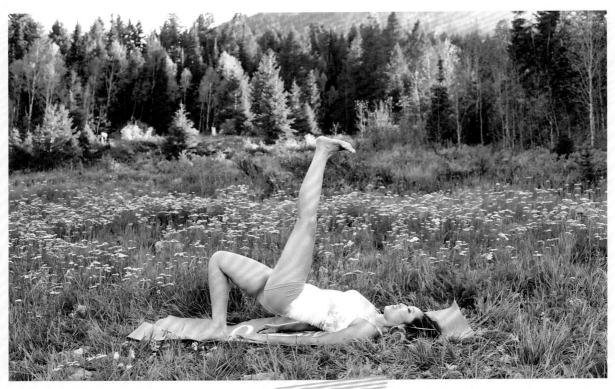

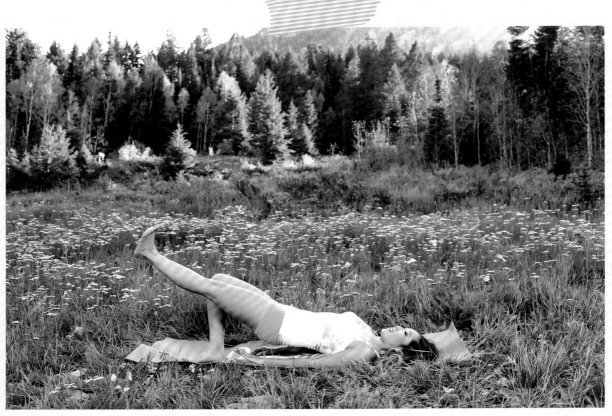

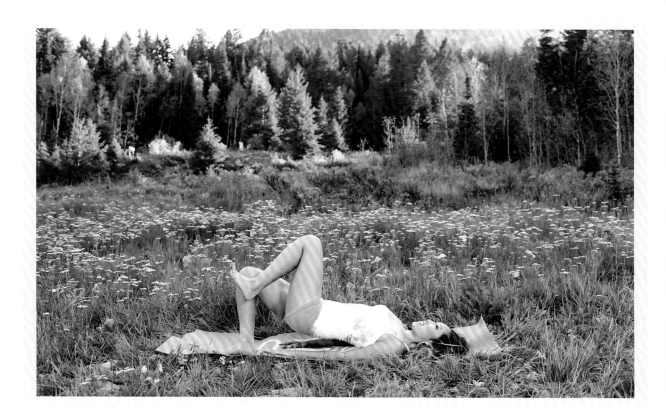

Feeling Bloated?

Oh, that's never a good feeling. Here's how to de-puff. Drink several glasses of water a day to restore the sodium imbalance in your body so that it will give up fluids. This will also help your system flush itself while keeping your digestive tract moving, thereby avoiding constipation. Also, don't skip your workout! This will help the gasses in your body from getting stuck.

SINGLE-LEGGED BIKE BRIDGE X 15 EACH LEG
WORKS: GLUTEUS

A Begin in Bridge with your upper back on the mat, hands relaxed and outstretched toward your hips, pelvis and glutes up in the air, knees bent, feet flat.

B Lift your left leg straight into the air perpendicular to the mat, foot flexed. Keeping your glutes lifted, drag your heel toward the mat and draw your knee toward your hips in a "bike pedaling" motion. That's 1 pedal. Repeat!

WORKOUT #3: LONG AND LUSCIOUS LEGS

Show off your stems this spring! Tighten and tone from calf to core with specialized workouts for firm, lean legs. These moves are sure to burn, but you'll feel cool as a cucumber strutting in your favorite sundress.

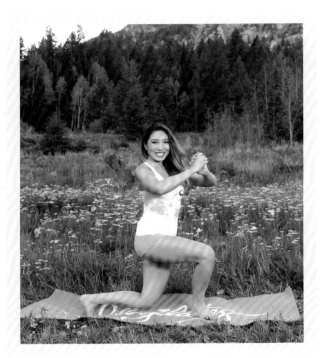 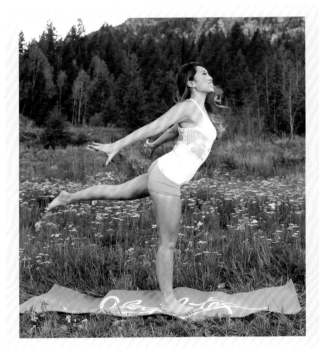

LUNGING BIRD X 10 EACH LEG
WORKS: QUADS, GLUTEUS, LOWER BACK

A Standing tall, bring your left leg behind you into a lunge. Both knees should be at 90-degree angles.

B Push off the ball of your left foot and raise your left leg into an arabesque with your arms stretched out behind you.

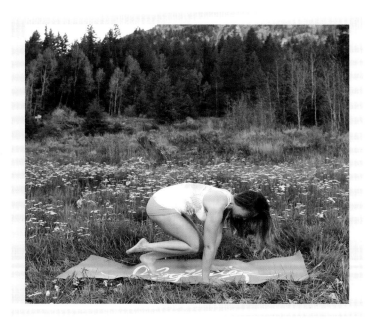

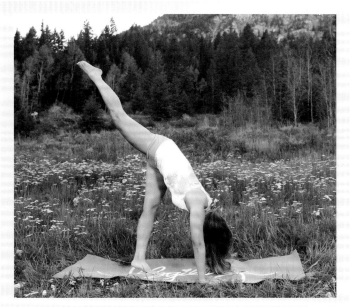

CALF ATTACK X 10
EACH SIDE
WORKS: CALVES

A Begin on the balls of your feet in a hunched-over position, chest to knees, hands flat on the mat, heels up. Bring your right knee into your chest and lift your right heel off the mat. In one motion, extend your right leg straight up into the air as high as you can go and straighten your left leg while keeping that heel up.

B Return to hunched-over knee-in position.

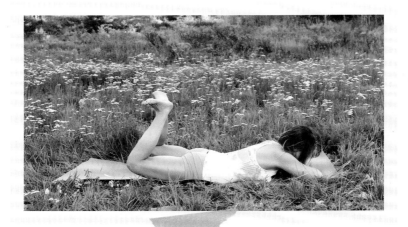

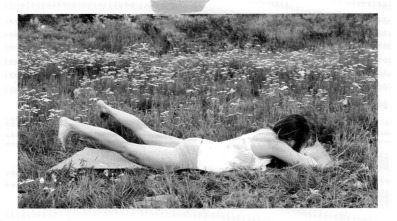

HAMSTRING KICKBACK
X 20
WORKS: HAMSTRINGS

A Lie on your belly, hands underneath your chin, chest resting on mat. Elevate your quads off the mat and flex your feet long behind you.

B Kick your heels to your butt, then extend them back out, all while keeping your quads off the mat. Beginners, if this is too difficult, simply start by keeping your quads on the mat.

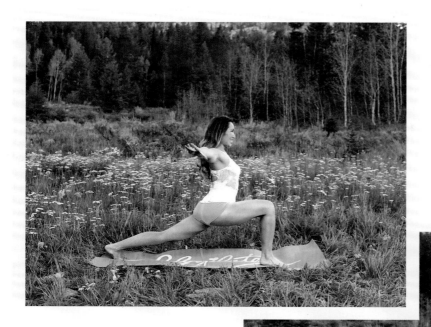

LONG LUNGE PULSE
X 10 EACH SIDE
WORKS: GLUTEUS, QUADS

A Begin by standing; bring your right leg in front of you and extend your left leg long behind you, knees straight, weight on the ball of your left foot. Your right leg should be at a 90-degree angle, foot flat. Hold the crown of your head high and make sure your hips are facing forward. Beginners, you may place your hands on top of your knee for support.

B Keeping your head at the same height at all times, bend your back knee to touch the mat; then, extend it to straighten the leg. Beginners, you do not need to touch the knee to the mat—just go as low as you can.

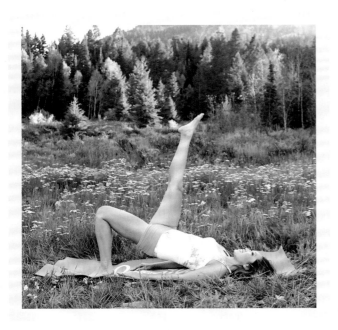

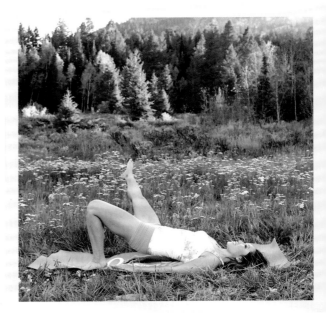

TRIANGLE BRIDGE
X 12 EACH SIDE
WORKS: GLUTEUS

A Begin in Bridge, with your hips elevated and your upper back pressed against the mat with your right leg pointed straight into the air.

B Draw a triangle with your toes while keeping your hips as steady as possible.

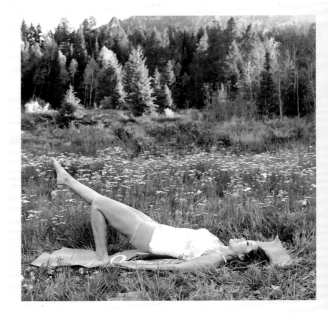

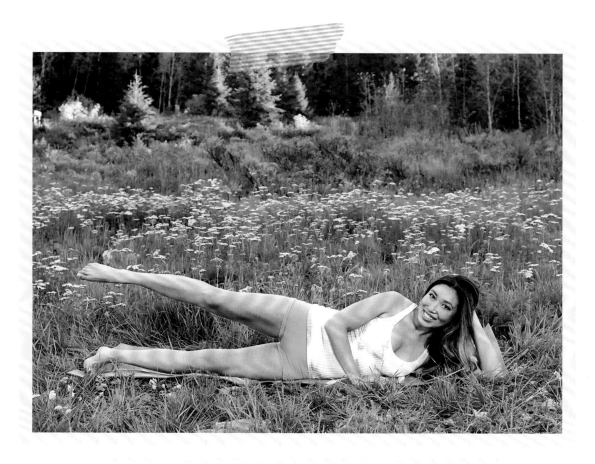

SIDE-LYING LEG CIRCLES X
12 FORWARD, 12 BACKWARD, EACH LEG
WORKS: INNER THIGHS, OUTER THIGHS

A Place one hand underneath your head and one in front of you to support your chest with your body long against the mat. Raise your upper leg high into the air and inhale as you bring the leg down in front of you.

B Exhale as you push your leg behind you, to close that circle motion. To make the move more advanced, widen your circle as big as you can while keeping your hips forward!

WORKOUT #4: UPPER BODY: TANK-TOP ARMS

Get tank-top ready with these all-encompassing upper-body exercises. You'll be firming up your chest, triceps, biceps, shoulders, and back, all the while aligning your body for better posture so you can enter spring feeling poised and confident.

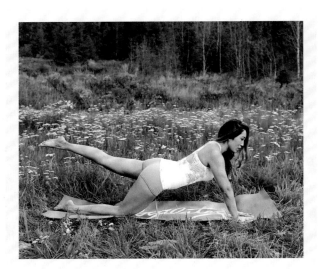 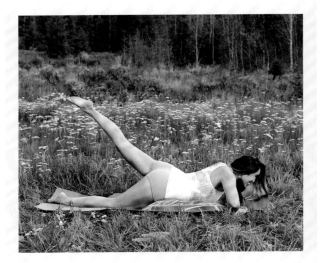

SINGLE-LEGGED TRIANGLE PUSH-UP
X 10 EACH LEG
WORKS: CHEST, TRICEPS

A Place your hands in a triangle position (thumbs and pointer fingers touching) on the mat slightly in front of your chest. Your back should be flat and angled downward as your left leg is extended behind you at the same height as your back. Beginners, you may keep both knees on the mat.

B Inhale and bring your chest as close as possible to the mat; exhale and press back to start position.

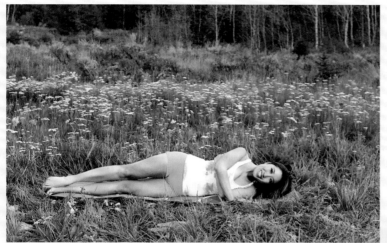

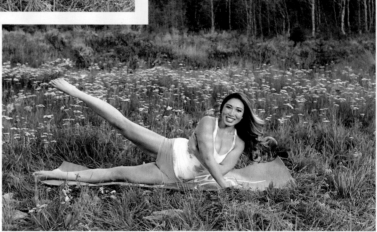

HUGGING SIDE SCISSOR X 12 EACH SIDE
WORKS: TRICEPS, PECTORALS

A Begin on your side, resting the side of your chest along the length of the mat. Bring your upper arm in front of you, heel of the palm pressed down into the mat. Your lower arm should caress your upper rib cage.

B Press all of your weight against your bottom hand and lift your chest off the mat. Return to start and repeat.

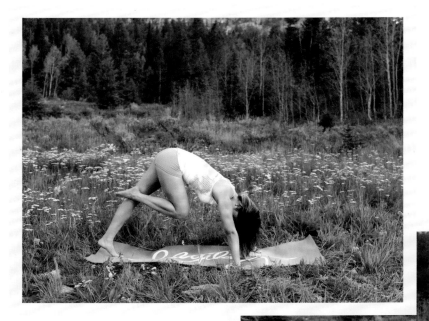

TUCKED SHOULDER PRESS
X 8 EACH LEG
WORKS: SHOULDERS, CORE

A Get into a Down Dog position with your heels pressed into the mat, palms flat, eyes toward the toes, and butt lifted into the air. Bring your right knee into the chest. Beginners, you may keep both your feet on the mat.

B Perform a Shoulder Push-up. Try to touch the top of your head to the mat while keeping your knee as close to your chest as possible.

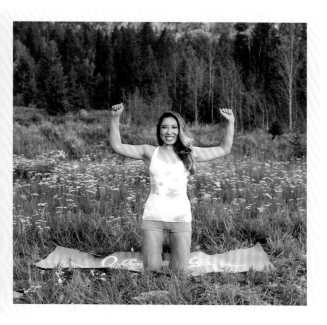

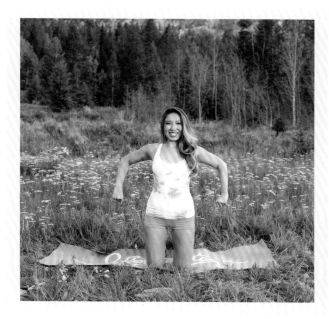

GOALPOST PUNCHER
X 20
WORKS: UPPER BACK, SHOULDERS

A Begin sitting tall with your arms raised at 90-degree angles like goalposts. Your legs may be crossed or in a Mermaid position to one side. Make sure to squeeze your shoulder blades together as if you're pinching something small, like a chestnut, behind your back.

B Leaving your elbows in place, bring your forearms down so that your arms are still at 90 degrees but upside down.

C Punch outward from your body with force.

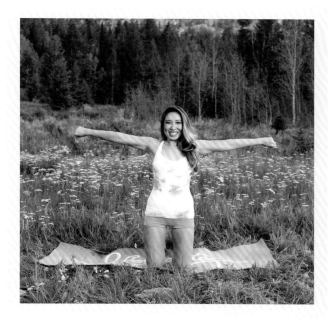

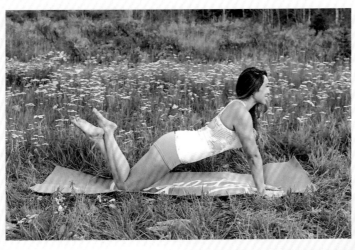

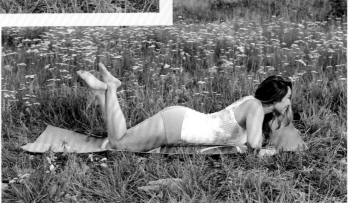

TRICEPS PUSH-UP X 12
WORKS: TRICEPS, CHEST

A Bring your hands into a triangle shape with your thumbs and pointer fingers touching. Your knees should be long behind you with your ankles crossed.

B Pushing through the heel of your palms, inhale and lower your chest as far as you can, then exhale and lift yourself back up as you straighten your arms.

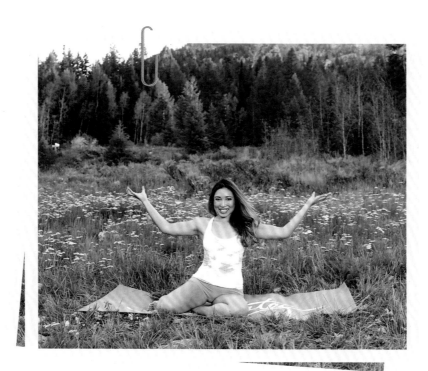

GOLF BALL X 50 FORWARD, 50 BACKWARD
WORKS: SHOULDERS, BICEPS, MENTAL STRENGTH

A Begin sitting, cross-legged or in a Mermaid position, with your legs to the side. Bring your arms out to the side with your elbows slightly bent and palms up, facing the sky, as if you are holding two golf balls.

B Do 50 mini circles forward, keeping the palms up! When you're done, do 50 back. Advanced students, you may repeat this for a second round but with "volleyballs"; try to keep the speed the same and keep your palms up—no stopping!

Too Sore?

That's a sign that you're using your muscles in a new way and they're not used to it! It's a bittersweet feeling that is painful—but good! If you're too sore to work out, then just focus on a different muscle group. If you simply need to rest (and that's totally okay), then make sure you drink tons of water to rehydrate your body. Take a hot bath to bring circulation to the sore parts. And be sure to stretch! You'll be back to good in no time.

WORKOUT #5: YOUR SPRING "LEANING" SLIM-DOWN

Slim down with this intense, total body workout that hits your obliques, abs, quads, core, and entire lower half. Kick it out—and stick it out—with the Burpee Kick, a super-hard, yet super-rewarding move. Give this one all you've got, and you'll love how you feel and what you see in the mirror.

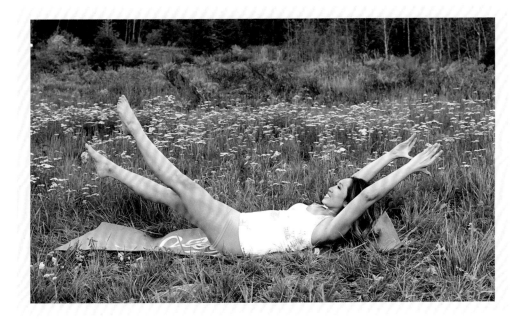

RUNAWAY ABS X 20
WORKS: CORE

A Place your hands long behind you, arms right by your head. Then, lift yourself into a boatlike position, head, neck, and shoulders up, hamstrings and legs off the mat straight in front of you. Your lower back should be pressed into the mat.

B Flutter your legs up and down, keeping your legs straight. Tighten your core and keep your arms behind you.

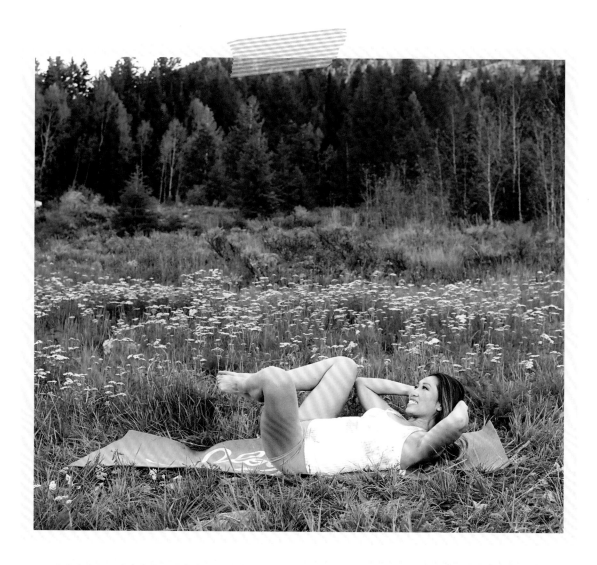

THE WIGGLE X 20
WORKS: OBLIQUES

A Bring your hands behind the nape of your neck, elbows wide. Then, bring your toes together, knees wide. Lift yourself up into Pilates Stance, meaning your head, neck, and shoulders should be lifted, eyes looking forward.

B Bring your right elbow to your right knee, then bring your left elbow to your left knee.

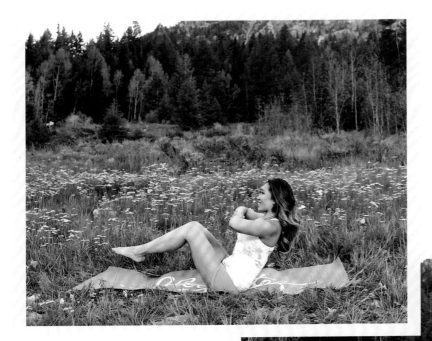

LEG-OUT X 20
WORKS: LOWER ABS, QUADS

A Bring your hands in front of you and clasp them together, elbows in a straight line. Balance yourself on your tailbone, knees together, feet together off the mat, back straight and tall. Beginners, you can leave your feet on the mat.

B Push your legs out in front of you, toes pointed, and exhale. Inhale as you bring your knees back in front of you. Beginners, you may push one leg out at a time with the other foot resting on the mat.

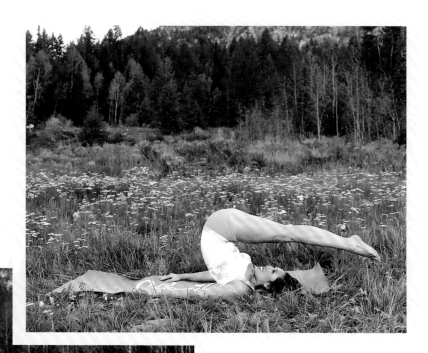

SQUATTING ROLLOVER X 12
WORKS: CORE, GLUTEUS, QUADS

A Lie with your back flat on the mat. Press your palms into the mat, press your heels together, point your toes, and tighten your abs as you lift your legs above your head. Beginners, you may use your hands to assist your lower back to get into the rollover position.

B Swiftly bring your legs forward in one sweeping motion, then hop your feet beside your hips, and position yourself in a squat. Beginners, you may simply land in a sitting position, feet right beside your body; then use your hands to assist yourself up into a squat.

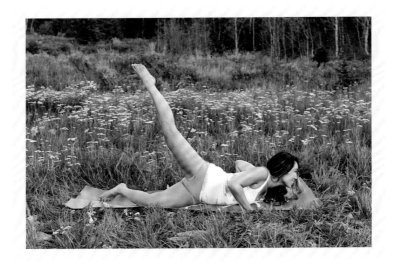

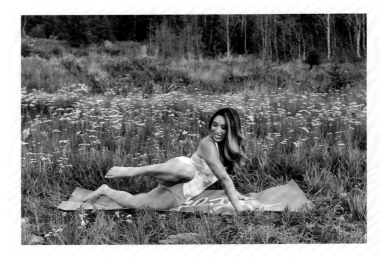

SADDLEBAG SHAVER X 12 EACH SIDE
WORKS: TRICEPS, CHEST, OUTER THIGHS

A Begin with your chest down on the mat, hands by your shoulders, elbows into your rib cage, left knee bent on the mat, and right leg extended long above you.

B Exhale and extend your arms until they are straight while bringing your right knee into your right elbow. Inhale and return to start.

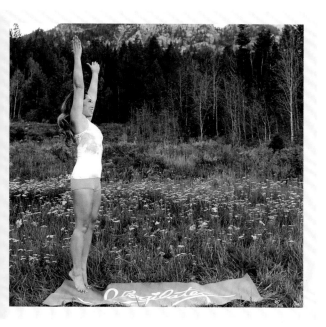

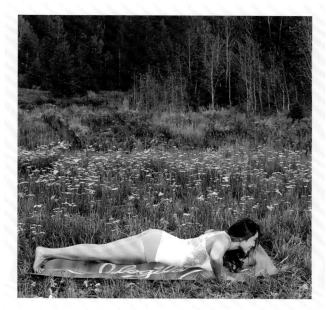

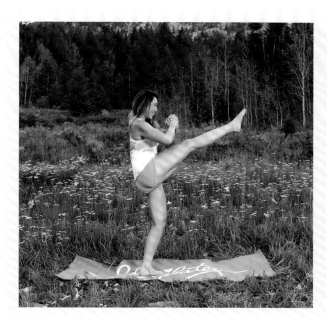

BURPEE KICK X 15
WORKS: TOTAL BODY, CARDIO

A Stand tall on the edge of your mat and perform a Burpee: jump high, then come into Plank as you land with your hands underneath your shoulders and your legs straight behind you. Make sure your lower back is flat and your hips don't sink! Do 1 push-up, then jump your feet in as close to your hands as possible and jump back up.

B Kick your right leg forward as powerfully as you can. Then kick your left leg. Start over!

A Note from Cassey

Unhappy with the Person I See in the Mirror

You look at yourself in the mirror and all you can think is: "I hate that stupid muffin top hanging over these stupid jeans that used to fit. Ugh. My arms look flabby. Eew. My abs are gone. My face looks puffier. Everything is just so **ugly**. How did I let this happen? I'm so fat. I hate myself. I hate my **life**!"

First of all, **Stop**. Stop the body shaming and stop using the word **fat** as a derogatory term. How much fat you have on your body has nothing to do with your self-worth! Stop torturing yourself with these insults!

Now listen.

I've had these days. Trust me. Being a fitness instructor doesn't mean you have immunity from gaining weight, being bloated, and feeling unmotivated. I, too, have looked in the mirror with an altered vision that could only pinpoint flaws. Both you and I need to stop judging ourselves and start loving ourselves. A body that is hated is one that will reject everything you want it to do. A body that is loved will respond positively.

It's important to understand that not every day will be one when you will see progress. In fact, you may train your butt off and eat clean as a bean for a week, but by Friday you may find that you've gained

5 pounds. And, you know what? It may not be 5 pounds of muscle, unfortunately.

It's called life.

The body is mostly predictable, but sometimes it's unpredictable. Yes, it's incredibly frustrating when you don't see immediate results from the hard work you've put in, but you must remember that as long as you're pushing forward and you're remaining focused, the changes you want to see in your body **will happen**. One day at a time.

However, you've got to be honest with yourself. Don't be slipping in junk foods, then complaining about why you don't see progress. A life of complaining, worrying, and not doing will lead nowhere.

If you're serious about getting that dream body and living the life you really deserve, then you've got to give yourself a fair chance. Give yourself 110 percent. Write down what you're eating, schedule your workouts, train seriously, and don't leave any tempting junk foods in the house. Create an environment that nurtures your success.

If you do this, I promise that you will enjoy the newfound control you have over your body and your health. **You are not a victim. Time does not control you. Food does not control you.** You are the one who decides how you want to feel and how you want to look. You'll radiate with confidence with this empowerment. I know it!

Remember to always love your body every step of the way.

♡ Cassey

SPRING EATS

Now for the spring foods! March, April, and May are so great because rain is filling the earth with the moisture it needs to grow a bountiful harvest of fruits and vegetables. Here are recipes that use those seasonal fruits and vegetables. For instance, the Mason Jar Bean Salad with Mango-Avocado Salsa (page 83) combines spring-harvested mango with avocado to fill your belly with the freshness of spring. And the fresh cherries in the Lemon-Cherry Quinoatmeal (page 82) give the quinoa bright flavors that are the perfect accompaniment to the spring's warming sun. And remember, you can play with your food to spruce up any ol' dish by exchanging it with whatever is freshly available.

SPRING'S IN-SEASON GROCERY LIST

Vegetables
artichokes
arugula
asparagus
Belgian endive
broccoli
butter lettuce
cauliflower
chives
collard greens
fennel
green beans
jicama
mustard greens
pea pods
radicchio
red leaf lettuce
rhubarb
snow peas
spinach
sugar snap peas
watercress

Fruits
apricots
grapefruit
limes
mangos
oranges
pineapples
strawberries

Sriracha Frittata

INGREDIENTS

1 teaspoon olive oil

½ red bell pepper, seeded and thinly sliced

¼ onion, thinly sliced

2 asparagus spears, trimmed and cut into ¼-inch slices

4 large egg whites

1 cup chopped fresh spinach (or baby spinach leaves)

2 teaspoons Sriracha hot sauce

DIRECTIONS

Preheat the oven to 375°F.

In a medium ovenproof skillet, heat the olive oil over medium heat. Add the red pepper and onion, and sauté for approximately 5 minutes. Add the asparagus and cook for another 3 minutes.

Whisk together the egg whites, spinach, and Sriracha in a bowl.

Pour the egg mixture over the vegetables in the skillet, and stir to distribute evenly. Cook until the egg mixture has set around the edges but is still a bit liquid in the middle.

Place the skillet in the oven for 10 to 12 minutes, or until the top is lightly browned and firm. Slice and serve.

149 calories, 5g fat, 13g carbs, 21g protein, 8g sugar

SERVES 1

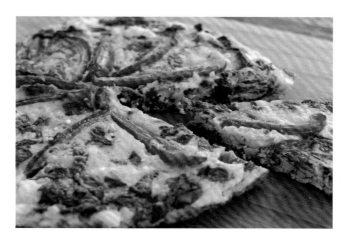

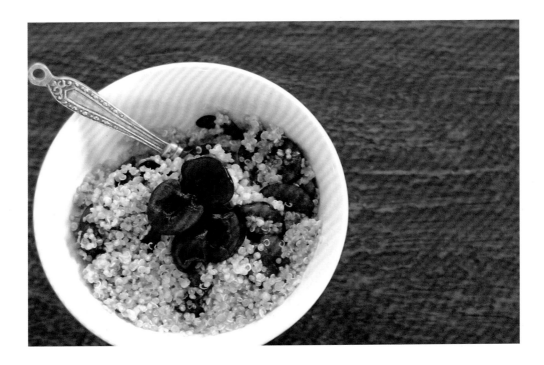

Lemon-Cherry Quinoatmeal

INGREDIENTS

¼ cup quinoa

¼ cup unsweetened almond milk

½ cup water

6 walnuts, chopped

¼ teaspoon grated lemon zest

Pinch of ground cinnamon

⅓ cup pitted and halved cherries

DIRECTIONS

In a medium saucepan, combine the quinoa, almond milk, and water and bring to a boil. Reduce the heat to low, cover, and simmer for approximately 10 minutes or until the quinoa is fluffy and the liquid is mostly absorbed. Fluff with a fork.

Fold in the walnuts, lemon zest, cinnamon, and cherries. Serve.

298 calories, 11g fat, 42g carbs, 9g protein, 11g sugar

SERVES 1

Mason Jar Bean Salad with Mango-Avocado Salsa

INGREDIENTS

- ½ cup cooked quinoa
- ¼ cup canned black beans, rinsed and drained
- ¼ teaspoon ground cumin
- ½ tablespoon fresh lemon juice
- Salt and pepper to taste

MANGO-AVOCADO SALSA

- ½ mango, flesh cut into cubes
- ¼ avocado, flesh cut into cubes
- ½ tablespoon fresh lime juice
- 2 tablespoons finely diced red onion
- 1 tablespoon finely chopped fresh cilantro

- ½ red bell pepper, seeded and chopped
- ¾ cup roughly chopped arugula

DIRECTIONS

Place the quinoa, beans, cumin, lemon juice, and salt and pepper in a pint-sized Mason jar. Close the jar with a lid and shake to mix.

Make the salsa: In a medium bowl, lightly toss the mango, avocado, lime juice, red onion, and cilantro.

Layer salsa on top of the quinoa mixture. Top with the red pepper and then the arugula. Serve.

379 calories, 10g fat, 67g carbs, 12g protein, 18g sugar

SERVES 1

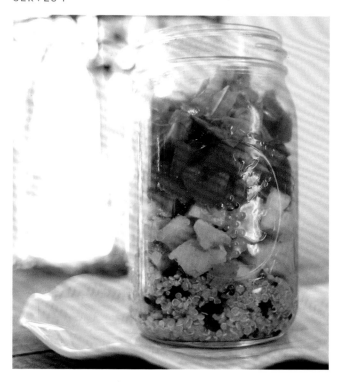

Veggie Burger

INGREDIENTS

2–3 tablespoons panko bread crumbs (or regular dried bread crumbs)

½ garlic clove, minced

½ cup canned black beans, rinsed and drained

¼ cup diced red bell pepper

Pinch of chili powder

½ teaspoon ground cumin

Salt and pepper to taste

1 tablespoon chopped fresh cilantro

2 teaspoons fresh lime juice

1 teaspoon olive oil

Whole wheat bun, toasted

Assorted toppings: mixed greens, tomato slices, nonfat Greek yogurt, mustard

DIRECTIONS

Place the bread crumbs, garlic, beans, red pepper, chili powder, cumin, salt and pepper, cilantro, and lime juice in a food processor and pulse until well combined.

Take the mixture out and shape into a patty.

Heat the olive oil in a medium nonstick skillet over medium-high heat. Add the patty and cook 3 to 4 minutes on each side, until nicely browned.

Place the patty on the bottom half of the bun and top with toppings of your choice. Add the top bun.

284 calories, 7g fat, 46g carbs, 13g protein, 5g sugar

SERVES 1

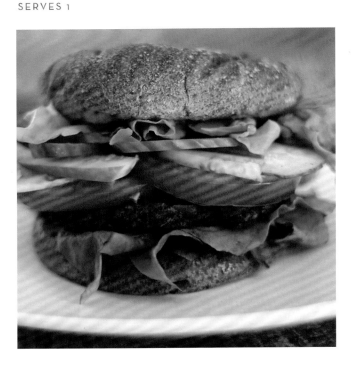

Tofu Stir-Fry

INGREDIENTS

1 tablespoon reduced-sodium soy sauce (or tamari)

½ teaspoon toasted sesame oil

1 tablespoon water

¼ block firm tofu, cut into cubes

⅓ cup sliced button mushrooms

¼ large red bell pepper, seeded and cut into strips

1 cup chopped broccoli florets

½ cup snow peas, trimmed

½ tablespoon reduced-fat peanut butter

2 cups chopped fresh spinach

½ cup cooked brown rice or quinoa

DIRECTIONS

In a nonstick skillet over medium heat, combine the soy sauce, sesame oil, and water. Add the tofu and simmer for 2 minutes. Add the mushrooms and raise the heat to medium-high. Cook for 5 minutes, stirring occasionally.

Add the red pepper and cook for 3 minutes. Add the broccoli, snow peas, and peanut butter and cook for an additional 2 minutes. Stir in the spinach and cook just until wilted, about 1 minute.

Serve over brown rice or quinoa.

253 calories, 10g fat, 30g carbs, 18g protein, 5.5g sugar

SERVES 1

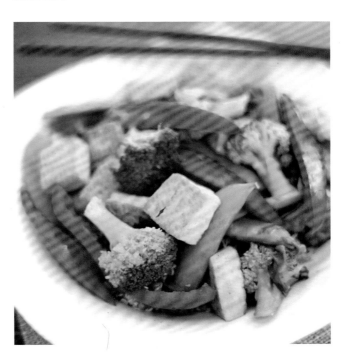

Chicken Parmesan

INGREDIENTS

- 1 (4-ounce) chicken cutlet
- ½ tablespoon prepared mustard
- Pinch of dried oregano
- 1–2 tablespoons grated Parmesan cheese
- Olive oil spray
- ½ cup low-sodium marinara sauce
- 2 cups chopped veggies of your choice (broccoli florets, zucchini, yellow summer squash, red bell pepper)

DIRECTIONS

Preheat the oven to 400°F.

Coat the chicken cutlet with the mustard, then sprinkle with the oregano. Pat the grated cheese on the chicken until it's well coated.

Spray a nonstick skillet with olive oil and place over medium-high heat. Sauté the chicken for 2 to 3 minutes on each side, until browned.

Mix the marinara and veggies in a bowl and pour into the bottom of a medium glass baking dish. Place the chicken atop the veggies and bake for 15 to 20 minutes, until vegetables are tender-firm.

312 calories, 12g fat, 17g carbs, 34g protein, 9g sugar

SERVES 1

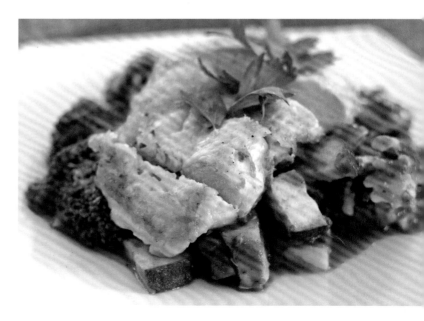

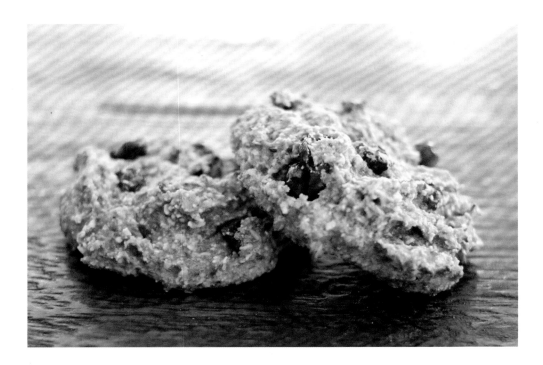

Orange-Cranberry Oatmeal Cookies

INGREDIENTS

Cooking spray

½ cup old-fashioned rolled oats

1 medium banana

1 teaspoon grated orange zest

1 tablespoon dried cranberries

DIRECTIONS

Preheat the oven to 350°F. Lightly coat a cookie sheet with cooking spray.

Place the oats, banana, and orange zest in a food processor. Process until well combined. Transfer to a bowl and carefully mix in the cranberries with your hands.

Shape the mixture into two cookies, and transfer to the cookie sheet. Bake for 15 minutes, or until the cookies are lightly browned and firm.

(for 1 cookie): 273 calories, 3g fat, 59g carbs, 6g protein, 19g sugar

MAKES 2 COOKIES

Shamrock Shake

INGREDIENTS

- 1 frozen banana
- 2 cups chopped fresh spinach
- ½ tablespoon agave nectar
- ⅛ teaspoon mint extract
- ⅓ cup water or coconut water
- ½ cup crushed ice
- 1 tablespoon dark chocolate chips (optional)

DIRECTIONS

In a blender, combine the banana, spinach, agave nectar, mint extract, water, and ice. Blend until smooth.

Stir in chocolate chips, if desired, and pour into a tall glass to serve.

182 calories, 4g fat, 40g carbs, 3g protein, 26g sugar

SERVES 1

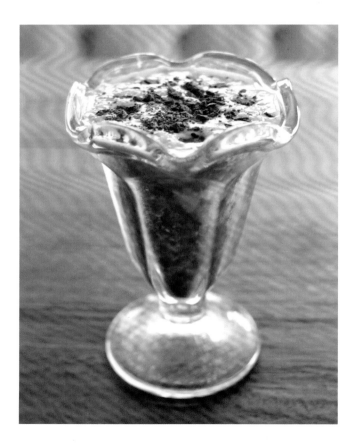

Piña Colada Protein Smoothie

INGREDIENTS

- 1 cup chopped frozen pineapple
- 1 cup coconut water
- ½ frozen small banana
- 1 scoop protein powder
- ½ cup crushed ice

DIRECTIONS

Place all the ingredients in a blender and blend until smooth. Pour into a tall glass and serve.

172 calories, .8g fat, 38g carbs, 6g protein, 31g sugar

SERVES 1

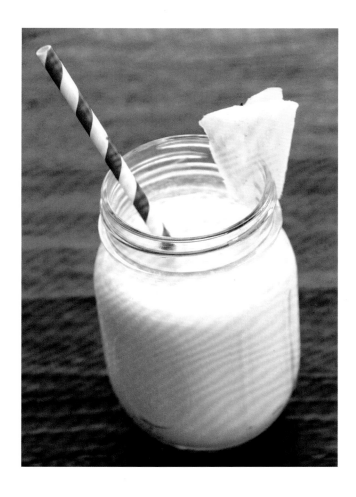

Spring Fast-Track Meal Plan

SUNDAY	MONDAY	TUESDAY	WEDNESDAY
Breakfast 1 cup cooked oatmeal, 1 apple	**Breakfast** 4 scrambled egg whites served atop 1 slice whole wheat toast with ¼ of an avocado spread on top	**Breakfast** Sriracha Frittata (page 81)	**Breakfast** Berry oatmeal: 1 cup cooked oatmeal mixed with ¾ cup sliced strawberries and 1 teaspoon agave nectar
Snack Plain 2% Greek yogurt	**Snack** Fresh Tacos (page 29)	**Snack** 1 ripe peach, 10 almonds	**Snack** Shamrock Shake (page 88)
Lunch Mexi-quinoa salad: ½ cup cooked quinoa, ¼ cup canned black beans, 2 cups chopped spinach, ½ cup pico de gallo	**Lunch** Turkey hummus wrap: 4 ounces low-sodium turkey slices, 2 ripe tomato slices, 1 cup mixed greens, wrapped in whole wheat tortilla that's been spread with 1 tablespoon hummus	**Lunch** Mason Jar Bean Salad with Mango-Avocado Salsa (page 83)	**Lunch** Chicken salad: 4 cups mixed veggies/lettuce (chopped tomato, cucumber, broccoli florets, bell peppers) and 1 (4-ounce) chopped cooked chicken cutlet, drizzled with vinaigrette of 1 tablespoon balsamic vinegar, 1 teaspoon olive oil, and ½ tablespoon lemon juice
Snack 10 carrot sticks, 2 tablespoons hummus	**Snack** 2 fresh apricots, 10 almonds	**Snack** Plain 2% Greek yogurt	**Snack** 2 Persian cucumbers, sliced, with 2 tablespoons hummus
Dinner Jolly green chicken: 1 (4-ounce) grilled chicken cutlet, served with mix of 1 chopped ripe tomato, 4 steamed asparagus spears, and ⅓ cup steamed chopped zucchini, dressed with 1 tablespoon chopped fresh basil and 2 teaspoons balsamic vinegar, topped with ¼ cubed avocado	**Dinner** Tofu Stir-Fry (page 85)	**Dinner** Fajitas: 1 (4-ounce) chicken cutlet chopped and sautéed with slices of ½ yellow and ½ red bell pepper, sliced onion, 1 chopped ripe tomato, 1 minced garlic clove, and a pinch of chili powder and ground cumin, served on a whole wheat tortilla	**Dinner** Chicken Parmesan (page 86)

Recipes with page references are included in this book; others are quick and easy to put together in a flash!

THURSDAY	FRIDAY	SATURDAY
Breakfast Lemon-Cherry Quinoatmeal (page 82)	**Breakfast** Plain 2% Greek yogurt with 1 cup mixed berries	**Breakfast** Spinach scramble: 4 large egg whites scrambled with 1 cup chopped fresh spinach and 1 tablespoon grated Parmesan, 1 slice whole wheat toast
Snack 1 cup pineapple cubes, 8 cashews	**Snack** 1 large hard-boiled egg, ¼ avocado	
Lunch Veggie Burger (page 84)	**Lunch** Chicken salad: 4 cups mixed veggies/lettuce (chopped tomato, cucumber, broccoli florets, bell peppers) and 1 (4-ounce) chopped cooked chicken cutlet, drizzled with vinaigrette of 1 tablespoon balsamic vinegar, 1 teaspoon olive oil, and ½ tablespoon lemon juice	**Snack** Orange-Cranberry Oatmeal Cookies (page 87)
Snack Fresh Tacos (page 29)		**Lunch** Mason Jar Bean Salad with Mango-Avocado Salsa (page 83)
Dinner Tofu Stir-Fry (page 85)		**Snack** 1 apple, 1 tablespoon almond butter
	Snack Piña Colada Protein Smoothie (page 89)	**Dinner** Protein plate: 4 ounces protein of choice (turkey or chicken) sautéed with 6 asparagus spears, 2 cups chopped spinach, ½ cup broccoli florets, and 1 tablespoon balsamic vinegar
	Dinner Fajitas: 1 (4-ounce) chicken cutlet sautéed with slices of ½ yellow and ½ red bell pepper, sliced onion, 1 chopped tomato, 1 minced garlic clove, and a pinch of chili powder and ground cumin	

A Note from Cassey

How to Motivate Yourself

Sometimes you just don't feel like it. I know, it's hard to move yourself off your bed or chair because you're thinking, **"Ugh, what's the point?"**

It's tough to get the ball rolling when it's been sitting idle for a while—well, at least that's when I feel least motivated to work out. It's not that I'm tired, it's just that I've been so out of the loop that everything feels rusty. This is the most uncomfortable part of motivating yourself. You feel lazy, slow, and weak. But sometimes you've just got to fight the discomfort until it gets better. You just have to. Don't whine. Put on your gym clothes, grab your water bottle, and **just go**.

Once you're back in the game, you'll get that exercise high, you'll see that strength coming back into your muscles, and you'll notice the incredible results. Personally, I think that results are the most motivating factor for me. They are the product of hard work and determination. It doesn't come easy, but nothing worth working for does, right?

If you're feeling sluggish, push that aside and just get out and work it. You know this is good for your body, so just do it. Stop thinking. I'm telling you to go **right now**. Sore today, strong tomorrow.

♡ Cassey

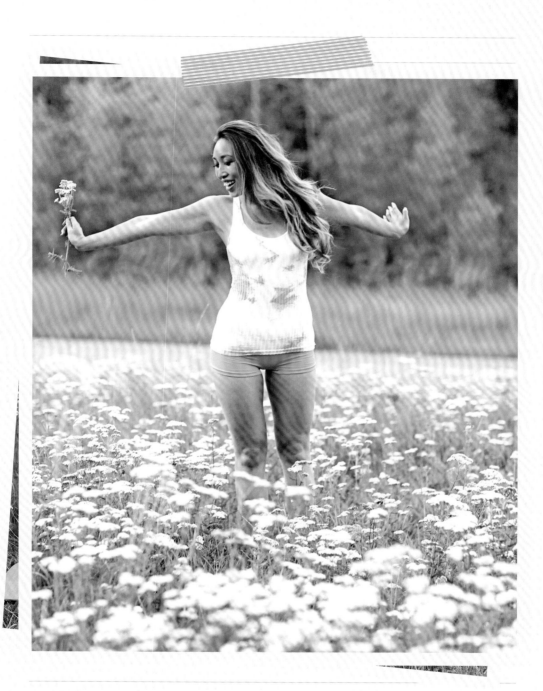

SUMMER

Summer

staying healthy during the active months!

This is the season of skin, sun, bikinis, and berries! Summer is my favorite time of year because the days are longer and brighter, giving me more time to play outside. As you start to peel off the layers of clothing, though, you may start to get hyper-conscious of your body. Though physical confidence is important, you must not forget that true beauty glows from the inside—from loving your body.

Summer is great because there are so many activities that keep you moving—swimming, hiking, biking down a path with the warm air racing through your hair, picnicking, especially with a basket of salads from the farmer's market! Since you're not in school right now, or your workplace might have shorter hours, it is easier to embrace these free days and schedule some exhilarating things to do. And while you're at it, bring those friends along who are also excited about breaking a sweat. You can even do group workouts in fun places like the beach or the park.

SUMMER MOVES

Keep in mind that one benefit of exercise (besides having flat abs or trim thighs) is that it can motivate you to work harder. How about being able to hold that Plank for 30 seconds longer than you did two weeks ago? How about being able to do more crunches than your boyfriend? How about feeling stronger? Feeling powerful? Being UNSTOPPABLE?

You'll notice I focus a lot on getting your body in shape for your bathing suit, targeting those areas that often make us cringe when we step onto the sand and reveal our body for the first time since last summer. Now, no one is perfect. Look around and you will quickly see that. But what you'll notice more are the men and women who are having the time of their lives, despite little dimples on the bum. I encourage you to build a healthier body—and know that you can achieve that goal if you work 110 percent during every workout.

Furthermore, I really want you to work hard this summer on something nonphysical. There will be days when you look in the mirror after weeks of exercise and you won't see those abs showing through. At this moment, you may feel like quitting. But you cannot get down on yourself. You did not fail. No. It's during these challenging moments that you must remember there is a bigger reason for putting yourself through all of this pain. You are stronger than you were on day one, and no one can take that away from you. Keep going, and everything will fall into place: a beautiful body and contagious confidence.

SUMMER, HERE WE COME!

WORKOUT #1: BIKINI AB ATTACK

Approve every bikini selfie you take this summer with this crazy hard ab workout. The Richter scale won't know what hit it, as your entire body shakes during the Earthquake move, but stay strong—you'll be beaming with confidence afterward and your beauty will glow from the inside out!

How to Look Slimmer and Taller Instantly!

Walk with your shoulders away from your ears and your chest held proud. This allows the neck to appear lengthened and elegant. Then, to create an instantly slimmer midsection, simply suck your belly button into your spine and wear a dress that cinches at the waist. Black is a universally slimming color. Finish with a pair of high heels to make your calves look strong and sexy. This combo will have you looking fabulous and, more important, feeling confident!

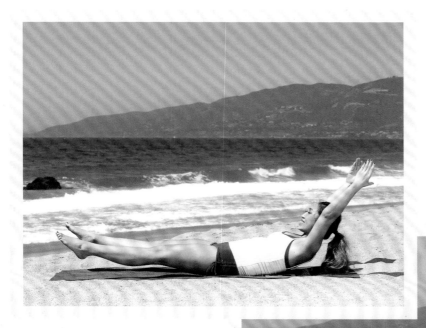

STAR ABS X 15
WORKS: ABS

A Lie like a star with your back on the mat and your arms outstretched long behind you, legs in front of you. Lift yourself into Pilates Stance, meaning head, neck, and shoulders lifted off the mat, abs engaged, eyes forward.

B In one sweeping motion, sit your whole body up onto your tailbone and hug your knees. Beginners, you can simply crunch and hug your knees while still lying on your back. Then return to start and don't rest your head on the mat.

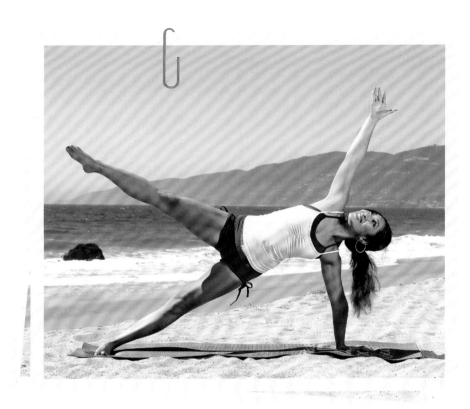

STARFISH SIDE PLANK FOR 30 SECONDS EACH SIDE X 2
WORKS: OBLIQUES, SHOULDERS, LEGS

A Lie on one side and place your bottom hand directly below your shoulder, your legs stretched long with your feet stacked on top of each other. Lift yourself up into a Side Plank. Beginners, you may stack your knees instead of your feet; you may also balance yourself on your elbow instead of your palm.

B While holding the Side Plank position, lift your upper leg as high as you can. Hold! Repeat for 30 seconds, two times on each side.

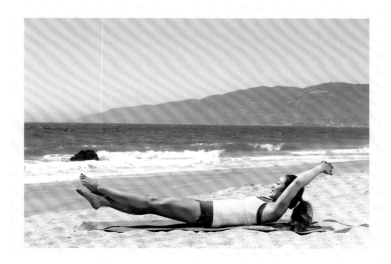

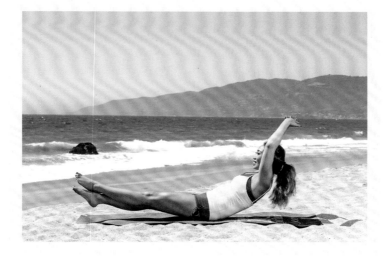

HOLLOW ROCK FOR 30 SECONDS X 2
WORKS: CORE

A Lying on your back, place your arms up above your head like a ballerina and cross your ankles, your legs straight in front of you.

B Pull your whole body up so that it represents the bottom of a boat with your tailbone and lower back against the mat only. Then, start rocking forward and back!

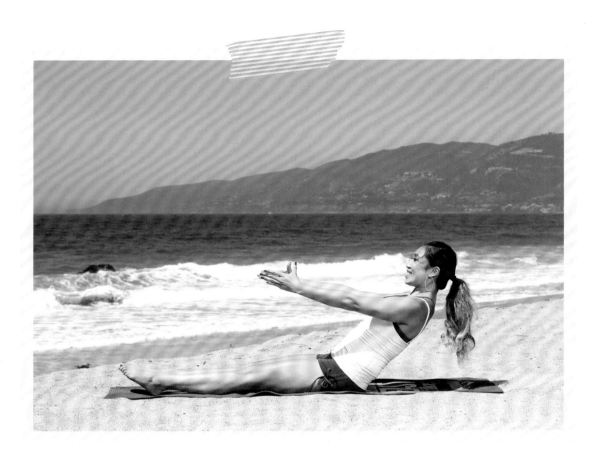

EARTHQUAKE X 15 SECONDS, 20 SECONDS, 30 SECONDS
WORKS: CORE

A   Sit tall with your legs touching side by side and pointed in front of you. Bring your arms long in front of you, parallel to your legs. Beginners, you may bend your knees and slightly curl your lower back into a Pilates C-Curve.

B   Lean back to your tipping point—right before you're about to fall backward and just holding on with the strength of your core. Hold. You will shake. That's why it's called Earthquake. To make the move more advanced, raise the arms to a diagonal. If you really want to increase the intensity, raise the arms directly above your head.

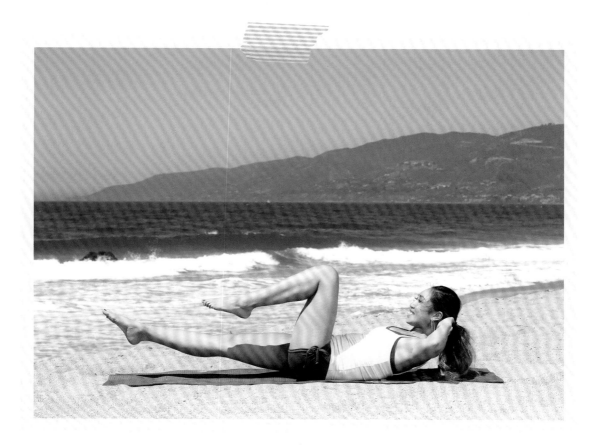

1-2-3 PULSE X 20
WORKS: LOWER ABS, UPPER ABS

A Bring your knees into Tabletop position, meaning knees bent at 90 degrees parallel to the floor, with your head, neck, and shoulders lifted into Pilates Stance, eyes looking forward. Your arms should be by your sides and reaching forward.

B Point your right leg out (1), then switch and point your left leg out (2), switch and point your right leg out again (3). Pause your legs here and do a mini crunch.

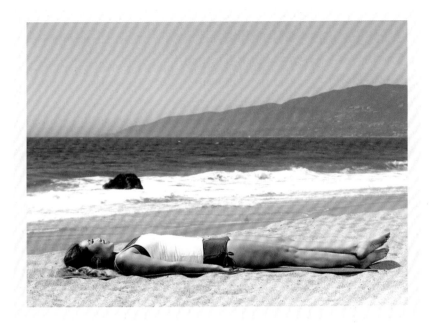

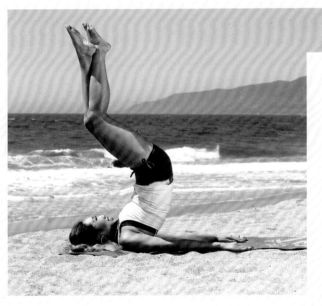

REVERSE CRUNCH
X 15
WORKS: LOWER ABS

A Lie with your back on the mat and your hands pressed down by your sides, head resting on the mat. Cross your ankles and place your knees in Tabletop position, meaning knees bent at 90 degrees parallel to the floor.

B Squeezing your lower abs, lift your tailbone off the mat and reach your toes to the sky!

How to Stay Active While Traveling

PACKING: Be sure to pack your sneakers, socks, and fitness clothes! This will encourage you to work out. No excuses.

ON THE PLANE: Try to get an aisle seat. This will allow you to take mini strolls when you start feeling cramped. You can also get up and do calf raises to wake up your legs. Try three sets of 12 to 15 each.

IN THE HOTEL: Always ask the front desk where the fitness center is. This way you'll be familiar with what the hotel has to offer. But if your place does not have one, I absolutely LOVE going for runs in a new city. It's the best way to tour your new destination while getting a workout! And if it's raining or you can't get outside, POP Pilates can always be performed in a small space like your hotel room.

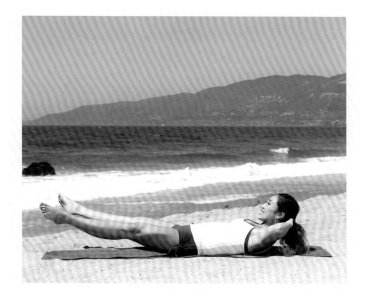

FLUTTERS X 20
WORKS: LOWER ABS, UPPER ABS

A Place your hands underneath the nape of your neck, elbows wide. Lift yourself into Pilates Stance, meaning your head, neck, and shoulders up, eyes forward. Bring your legs straight in front of you, elevated a few inches off the mat.

B Bring your feet out hip width apart, then in, tapping your heels together.

WORKOUT #2: BIKINI BOOTY BUILDER

Tighten and lift your derriere, and show it off at the beach. These Clamshell variations make your booty as sleek as a pearl. Turn up the music and release your inner dancer with the Dancer's Sweep for a poised and graceful silhouette.

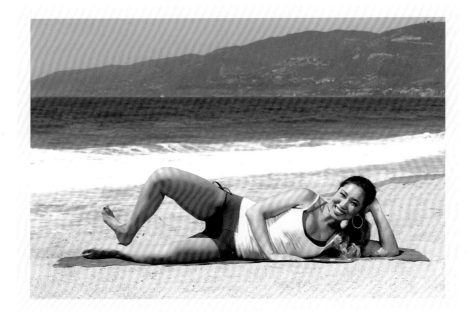

CLAMSHELL X 20 EACH SIDE
WORKS: GLUTEUS

A Lie down on your side and support your head with your bottom hand. Your upper arm should be resting in front of you, supporting your chest. Your knees should be in Fetal Pose, stacked on top of each other bent forward at about a 90-degree angle.

B Exhale and open the knees wide, keeping the chest forward and the heels glued together. Inhale down.

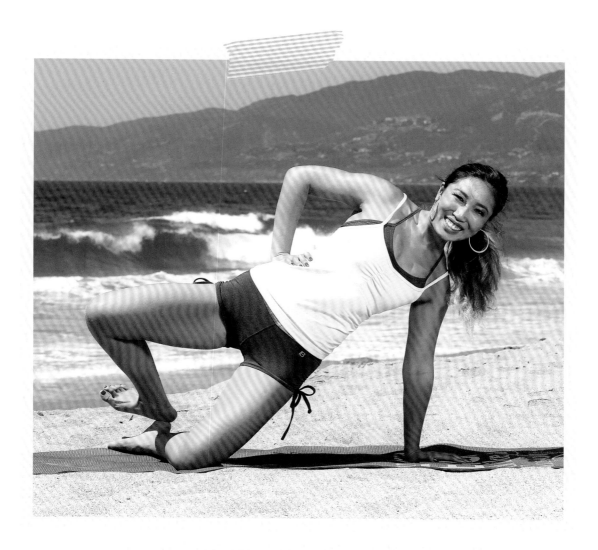

ELEVATED CLAMSHELL X 20 EACH SIDE
WORKS: GLUTEUS, OUTER THIGHS

A With your knees in Fetal Pose, elevate your upper body by placing your bottom hand underneath your shoulder and extending your arm straight. Your upper hand should be on your hip.

B Open your knees wide with the heels glued together as you exhale. Inhale down.

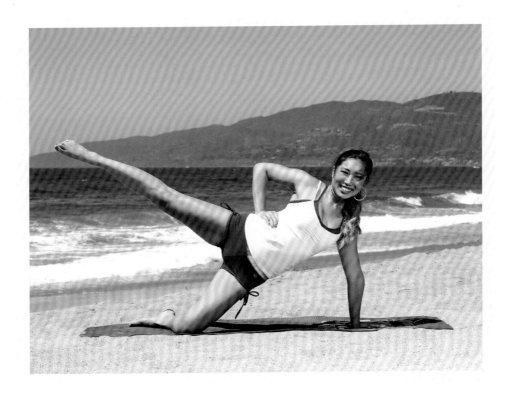

ELEVATED CLAMSHELL LEG LIFTS X 20 EACH SIDE
WORKS: GLUTEUS, THIGHS

A Place your bottom hand underneath your shoulder and your upper hand on your hip. Lift into a Side Plank with your bottom knee on the mat and upper leg extended long.

B Lift your top leg up and down. Exhale up and inhale down.

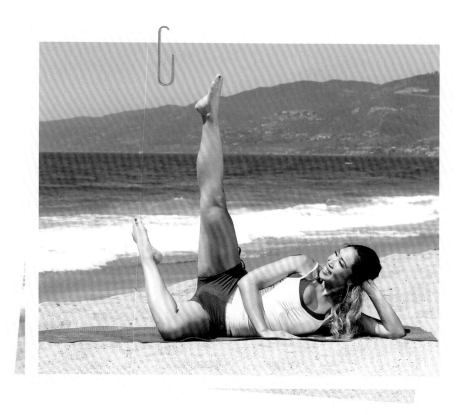

HALF CLAM CIRCLES X 10 FORWARD, 10 BACKWARD
WORKS: GLUTEUS, THIGHS

A Place your bottom hand underneath your head, your top arm in front of you, supporting your chest. Start with both legs in Fetal Pose, then raise your top leg as high as possible, toes pointed to the sky. Your bottom knee should be on the mat, bent forward, but toes up to the sky.

B Create mini circles with your top leg, going forward for 10 and then backward for 10. Switch legs when done!

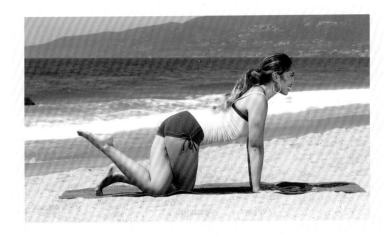

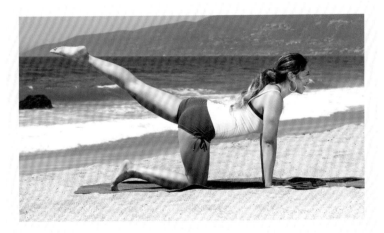

CROSS BUTT LIFT AND TAP
X 20 EACH SIDE
WORKS: GLUTEUS, THIGHS

A Get on all fours, hands underneath your shoulders, palms flat, knees hip width apart. Bring your left knee over your right and tap the mat.

B Extend and lift that left leg straight out behind you.

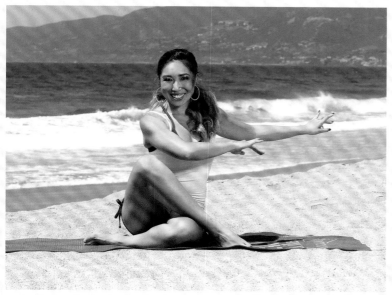

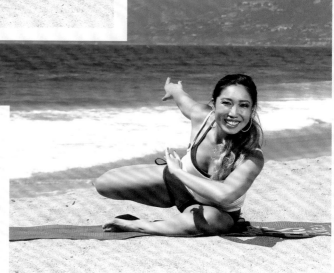

DANCER'S SWEEP
X 20 EACH SIDE
WORKS: GLUTEUS, LOWER BACK,
THIGHS

A Start with your left knee underneath you and your right knee crossed above, toes slightly touching the mat. You're in a pretty twisted position. Bring your arms all the way to the left side.

B Exhale and extend the right leg out in front of you, then circle it back to the right into an attitude, bowing your chest forward. Your arms should travel to the right as well. Inhale and bring back to start.

WORKOUT #3: SLIM SWIMSUIT THIGHS

Rock your short-shorts and miniskirts with superstar thighs. Focus here on your precision and form, and when you get the hang of it, see how fast you can go during the Elevated Hot Potato—challenge yourself through the burn!

FROGGERS X 15
WORKS: INNER THIGHS

A Place your hands behind your head, elbows wide, head, neck, and shoulders up in Pilates Stance, eyes forward. Flex your feet and place your heels together, knees super-wide right above the hips. Beginners, you may keep your head down, hands in a triangle underneath your tailbone.

B Exhale and push your heels forward like you're pushing a really heavy door open. Your legs will straighten and your knees will come together, but your heels must remain glued! Inhale back to start.

Don't Believe in Yourself?

Well, you should. Because I do. Your self-confidence is your biggest asset, and you should do everything you can to nurture it. Don't ever let small minds convince you that your dreams are too big.

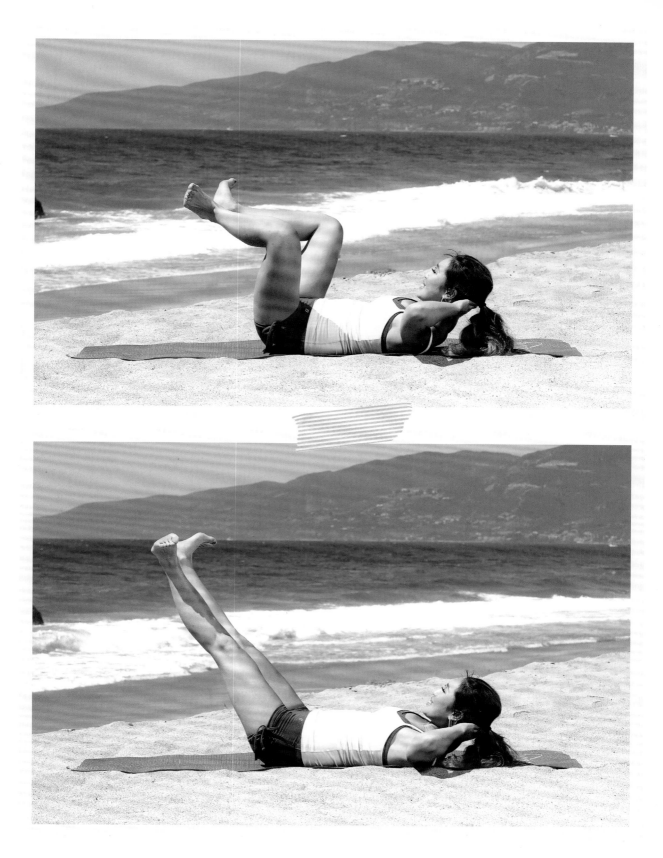

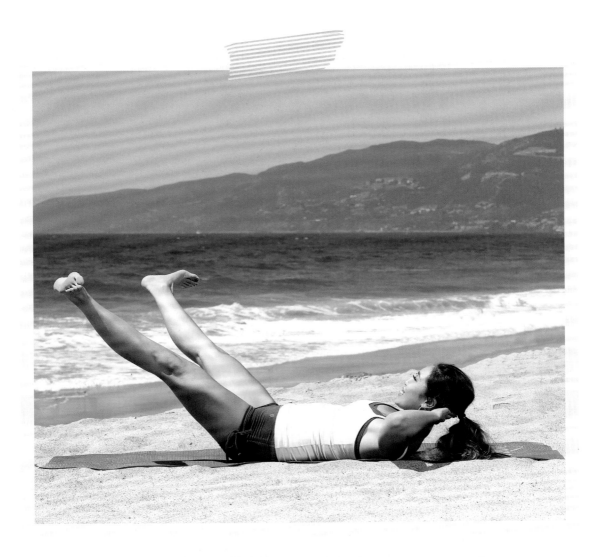

FROGGY HEEL CLICKS X 20
WORKS: INNER THIGHS, QUADS, LOWER ABS

A Bring your hands behind your head, elbows wide, head, neck, and shoulders up in Pilates Stance, eyes forward. Lift your legs up and out in front of you, feet flexed.

B Click your heels together while keeping your legs straight, in and out.

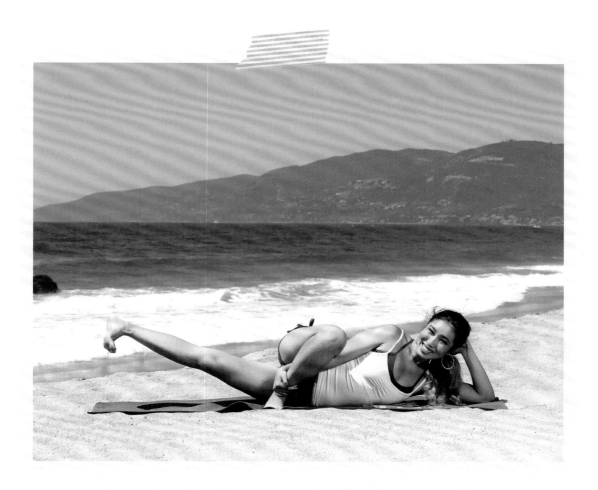

INNER THIGH LIFT X 20 EACH SIDE
WORKS: INNER THIGHS

A Lying on your side, place your bottom hand underneath your head, pull your upper leg and foot toward your chest, and hold your ankle with that top hand. Extend the bottom leg, and create an "awkward foot"—meaning heel up, toes down. This may feel a bit weird, but it will really help you target your inner thighs.

B Keeping that bottom leg straight, press your heel up into the air, foot flexed. Bring back down and repeat.

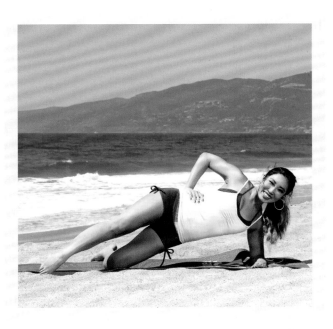

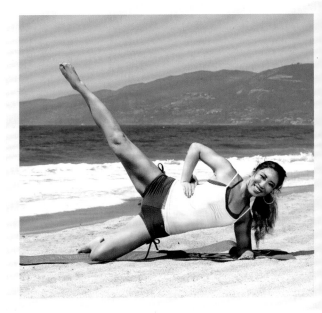

ELEVATED HOT POTATO
X 12 EACH LEG

WORKS: OUTER THIGHS, GLUTEUS

A On your side, support your head with your bottom hand and bring your upper arm on your hip. Stack your knees on top of each other, then extend your top leg out.

B Bring the top leg in front of you, keeping it straight, and "tap, tap" the mat in front of you, then lift up super-high and "tap, tap" behind you. You should be drawing a big triangle. Every time your leg reaches the top of the triangle, that counts as 1.

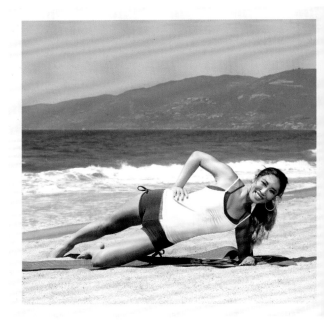

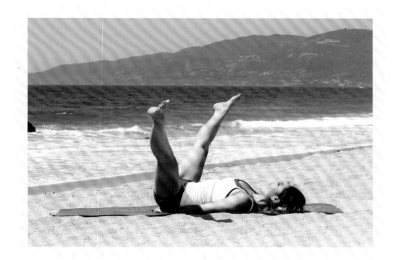

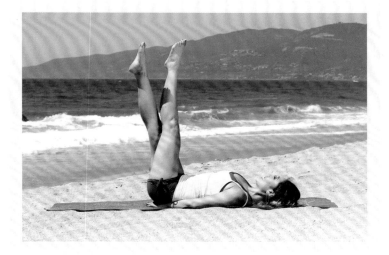

SIDEWAYS SCISSORS X 20
WORKS: INNER THIGHS, OUTER THIGHS, LOWER ABS

A Lie on your back and place both hands in a triangle right underneath your tailbone for support, head resting on the mat. Bring your legs straight up to the sky, toes pointed.

B Inhale, move your legs wide apart, then exhale and bring them back up, ankles crossed.

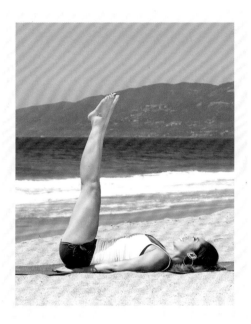

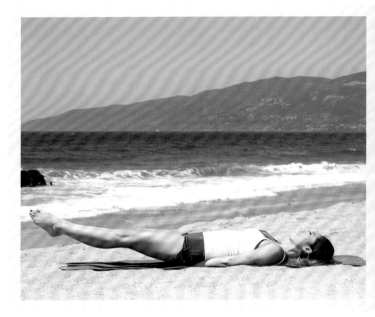

DOUBLE D'S X 12
WORKS: LOWER ABS,
THIGHS, QUADS,
HIP FLEXIBILITY

A Lie on your back and place both hands in a triangle underneath your tailbone for support, head resting on the mat. Bring your legs straight up to the sky, toes pointed. Make sure your lower back is pressed down into the mat.

B Inhale and bring your legs straight down, feet together. On the exhale, circle your legs outward and up. Imagine you're drawing two capital D's.

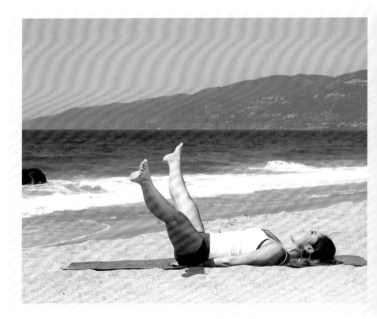

WORKOUT #4: PERKY CHEST AND SVELTE ARMS

We're going tropical with this workout by channeling our inner reptile, climbing our way up to chiseled chest and arms with The Gecko move, then lifting our bikini tops with the Pray 'n' Pulse—a deceivingly innocent move.

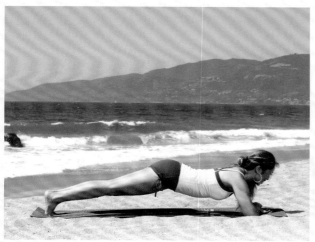

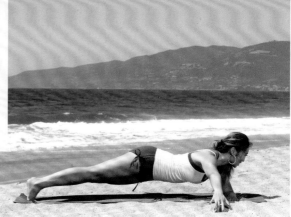

THE GECKO X 20 TAPS
WORKS: SHOULDERS, CORE, CHEST

A Begin in a Plank with your hips lifted, butt in line with the rest of your body, elbows crossed underneath you.

B Bring your right arm out to your right side and tap the floor with your fingers. Bring your right arm back to the crossed-arm position and extend your left arm to the left side, tap.

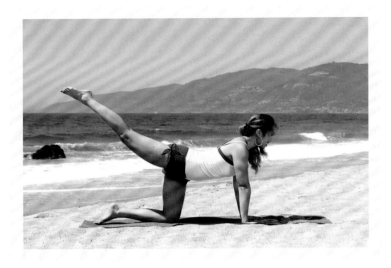

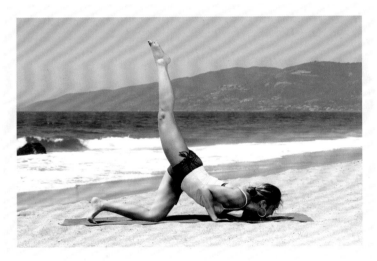

OIL RIGGER X 15 EACH LEG
WORKS: TRICEPS, CHEST

A Get on all fours with your palms underneath your shoulders, arms extended, knees hip width apart. Extend your right leg long behind you and lift as high as you can, toes pointed.

B Keeping your elbows close into your rib cage, inhale and perform a triceps push-up, bringing your chin forward and down touching the mat. Exhale and lift up.

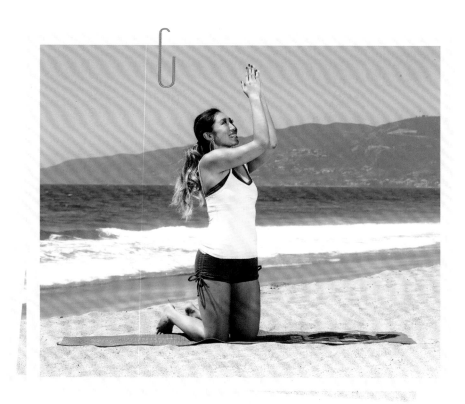

PRAY 'N' PULSE FOR
25 PULSES X 2 SETS
WORKS: PECTORALS, BICEPS

A Sit tall however you feel comfortable. Just make sure your back is straight and tall. Bring your elbows together and place your palms together as if you're praying.

B Bring your elbows up from shoulder height toward nose height. Never let your elbows come apart.

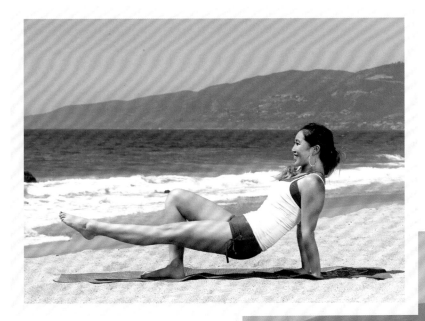

TRICEPS KICK 'N' DIP X
15 EACH LEG
WORKS: TRICEPS

A Facing up, balance yourself on the soles of your feet and your palms, your fingers facing toward your feet. Raise your left leg parallel to the mat.

B Inhale and bend your elbows to perform a triceps dip while kicking your left leg up. Exhale and return to parallel leg and straight arms.

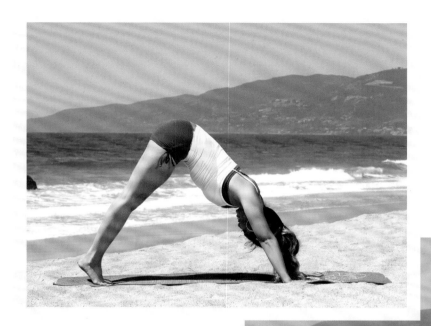

SHOULDER PUSH-UP X 12
WORKS: SHOULDERS

A Get into a comfortable Plank position, then raise your butt into the air and walk your hands back about two hands-lengths in. You should be in a Down Dog position.

B Keeping your eyes focused on your toes, inhale and press your head down toward the mat as your elbows bend outward. Exhale and straighten your arms.

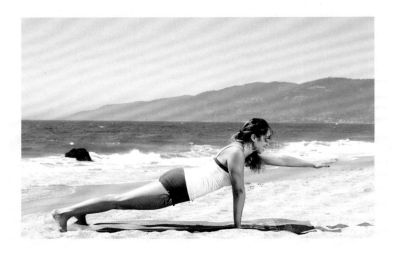

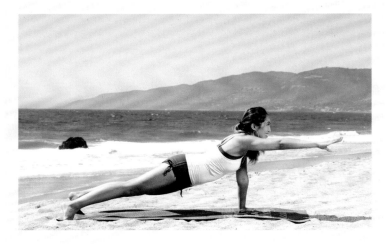

BEACH REACHES X 20
WORKS: CORE, CHEST, SHOULDERS

A Begin in Plank with your hands underneath your shoulders, arms straight, and feet hip width apart. Beginners, you may do this move on your knees.

B Keeping your hips square to the mat, raise your left arm forward, then your right, alternating. Hold for about 1 second when you reach forward.

A Little Friendly Motivation . . .

Sometimes a friend's dislike for physical activity and healthy eating is linked to her own insecurities. No need to make the friend feel bad; instead, slowly introduce her to your world and show her how much fun it can be. Ask your friend to come over for dinner and help you cook an eat-clean dish. After the meal, go for a walk and talk to burn off the calories while you catch up with what's happening. Next time, ask her to go shopping with you and trick your friend into the ever-inviting and amazingly bright fitness clothes section! She won't be able to resist! Then invite her to hang out at your place and see if she wants to work out with you. It's all about helping the people you care about find the joy in exercise. Once that's accomplished, she'll keep coming back.

WORKOUT #5: THE ULTIMATE SWIMSUIT SLIM-DOWN

Seduce your summer fling with this sizzling cardio routine. The Scorpion Push-up works every muscle in your body, twisting and turning for the ultimate fat-stinging workout.

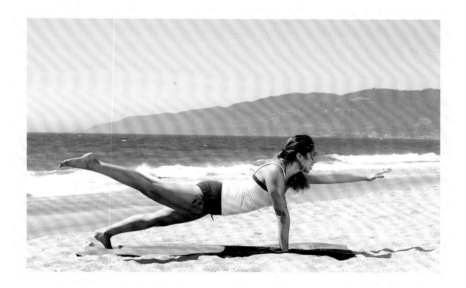

ADVANCED PLANK FOR 10 SECONDS EACH SIDE X 6
WORKS: CORE

A   Begin in a Plank position, hands underneath your shoulders, arms straight, and feet a little wider than shoulder width apart.

B   Keeping your hips in line with the rest of the body and square to the mat, lift your right arm and your left leg. Hold. This is very advanced. Beginners, you may start with Plank on your knees and lift the opposite arm and leg.

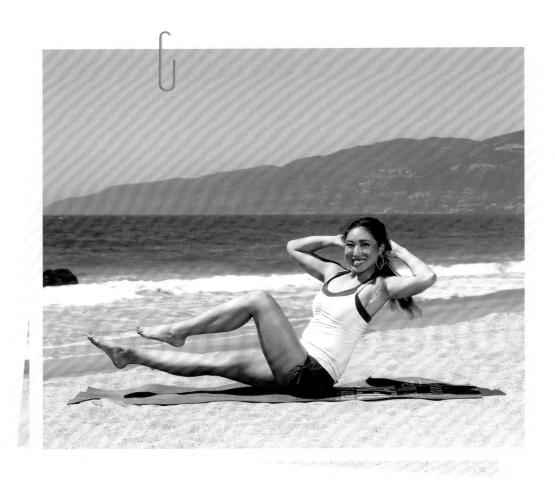

SEATED CRISSCROSS X 20
WORKS: OBLIQUES, QUADS

A Balance on your tailbone and sit tall with your knees up, toes pointed.

B Bring your right shoulder toward your left knee as you extend your right leg forward. Switch.

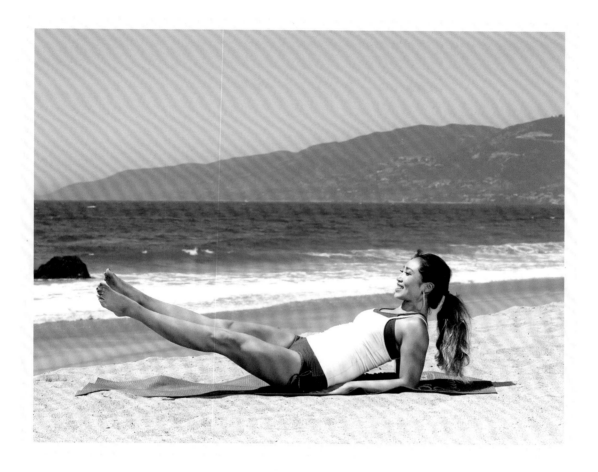

CLOCK ABS X 8 CLOCKWISE, 8 COUNTERCLOCKWISE
WORKS: LOWER ABS, QUADS

A Pretend you're sunbathing with your elbows behind you, fingers toward your feet, chest open. Then lift your legs straight up into a diagonal, heels pressed together, toes pointed. Beginners, you may keep the knees bent.

B Draw a circle with your toes as you go clockwise. Then stop on top and go counterclockwise. Beginners, you draw a circle with your knees.

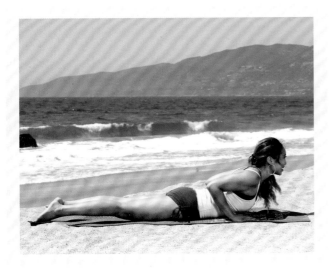

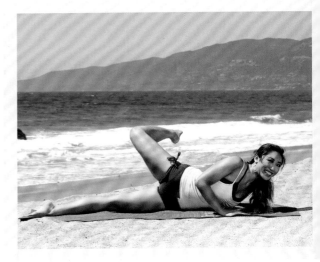

SCORPION PUSH-UP
X 20
WORKS: TRICEPS, CHEST, LOWER BACK

A Lie flat on your belly and bring your hands right beside your shoulders.

B Keeping your elbows into your rib cage, open up your right hip and knee and tap the right toe on the left side of your body as you twist the lower back. Your arms will perform a Triceps Push-up as you do this. Alternate sides, to count as 1 rep.

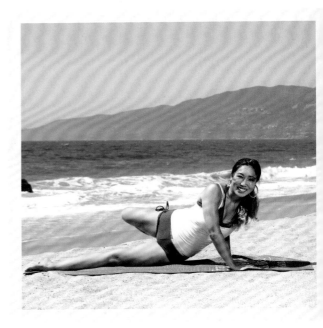

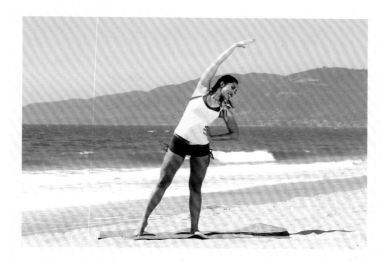

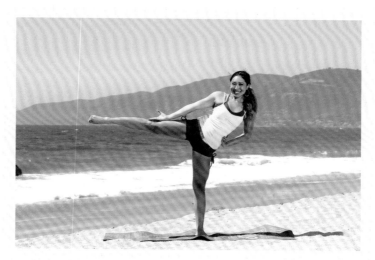

STANDING SIDE SQUEEZE X 15 EACH SIDE
WORKS: OBLIQUES, BALANCE

A Stand on your mat with your left hand on your hip, right leg stretched out to the side and right arm elegantly extended over your head like a ballerina.

B Exhale and bring your right arm to your right leg, keeping it straight and squeezing your obliques. Inhale back to start.

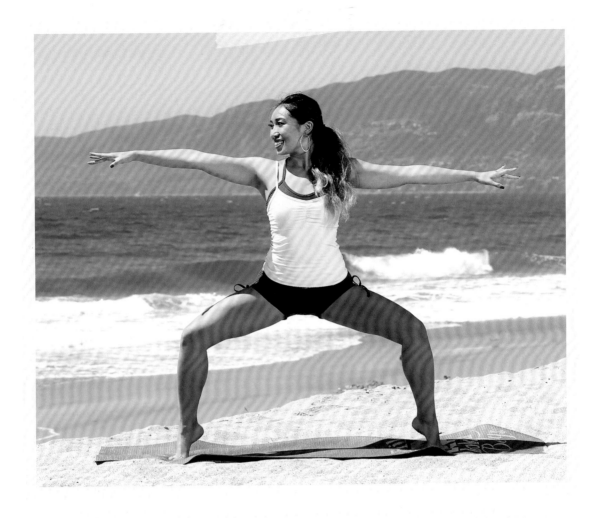

PLIÉ HEEL LIFTS X 25
WORKS: CALVES, QUADS, INNER THIGHS, GLUTEUS

A Bring your legs out much wider than shoulder width, with feet as parallel to the edge of your mat as you can. Beginners, you can bring your feet diagonal. Stretch your arms out to the side, shoulder height, fingers soft. Press your butt down into a Plié Squat and stay there.

B Lift your heels up, then drop them down while staying low in your Plié Squat.

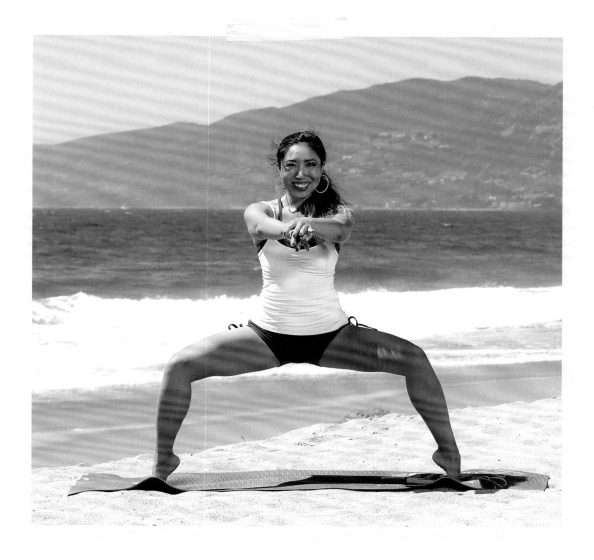

PLIÉ PULSES X 25
WORKS: GLUTEUS, QUADS, INNER THIGHS, CALVES

A Stay in your low Plié Squat position and keep your heels lifted, arms straight in front of you, hands clasped.

B Pulse your bottom down and up staying super low. Never straighten the legs.

A Note from Cassey

Happiness Is Not a Number

The pounds you lose are just one measure of your success. Yet, over and over again, many of us let our well-being be defined by the number we see between our feet. And it doesn't stop there. We confuse how much money we make or the number of bedrooms in our house with our self-worth. Magazines, TV shows, and movies tell us that beautiful models, married to rich businessmen, living in glamorous mansions, driving exotic cars, are the definition of success, but that's not true. Success is a state of being. Being happy.

Now, I'm not telling you to just sit and stop trying to lose weight or get a promotion. I'm telling you that you've got to see the difference between the milestones of success and self-worth.

As a human being, all I can ask from you is that you find your passions and live to realize your own honest potential. The key words here are **own potential**—not someone else's expectations. You're not here to compete with anyone else or to worry about how famous, how rich, or how skinny your friends are getting. Does it matter? What does that have to do with you?

If you work toward being the best version of you—every day—no one can even compare!

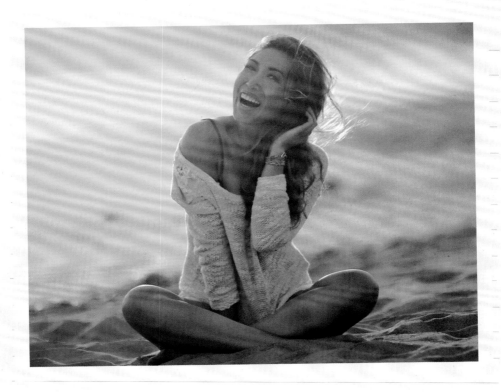

You've got to dive into your talents, make them shine, and share what you've got with everyone around you to improve and inspire better lives. Success isn't a destination, it's an enlightened state of being that starts with your own self-acceptance.

    I urge you to live life to your best abilities.

Live passionately and live purposefully. Live beyond a number. Beyond what people expect of you. Live to appreciate your own self-worth. When you do this, you will achieve anything and everything you've ever wanted. I see it in your future.

♡ Cassey

SUMMER EATS

Welcome to Salad Season, when veggies and fruits are everywhere, crazy to fill your plates with an abundance of clean eats! For the Pancakes with Berry Applesauce (page 133), I grabbed the prettiest raspberries on the shelf and created the most vibrant topping you'll ever see on pancakes, but you can also use blueberries or strawberries or blackberries—or go crazy and use them all! Again, it's about using what's fresh and having fun, so that you are motivated to replenish your body daily with the nutrients these fresh foods contain. I give you a lot of salad recipes for the summer because they are easy and cool. Since there are so many things that are sold fresh and ready for you to pick, have at it. Make the Summer Salad with Avocado Dressing (page 137) and Eggplant Enchilada Tower with Zucchini Salsa Verde (page 138) and see how the garden looks on your plate.

SUMMER'S IN-SEASON GROCERY LIST

Vegetables
arugula
beets
broccoli
butter lettuce
cucumbers
eggplant
endive
green beans
hot peppers
okra
radishes
red leaf lettuce
snow peas

sugar snap peas
summer squash
Swiss chard
tomatoes
zucchini

Fruits
apricots
Asian pears
blackberries
blueberries
boysenberries
cantaloupe

cherries
elderberries
figs
grapes
honeydew melon
limes
nectarines
passionfruit
peaches
pineapples
plums
raspberries
strawberries
watermelon

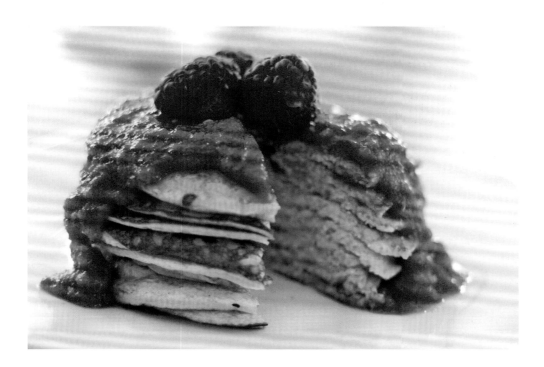

Pancakes with Berry Applesauce

INGREDIENTS

BERRY APPLESAUCE

½ apple, unpeeled, cored and diced

⅛ cup water

¼ cup raspberries (or strawberries, blueberries, blackberries, or mixed)

PANCAKES

2 large eggs

2 ripe bananas

Cooking spray

DIRECTIONS

Make the applesauce: Place the diced apple and water in a small skillet or saucepan. Cover and simmer over low heat for 6 to 8 minutes, until the apple is fork-tender. Turn off the heat and add the berries. Stir gently and allow to cool. Place in a blender and whirl until smooth. Transfer to a bowl.

Clean the blender jar and add the eggs and bananas, blending until smooth.

Coat a small skillet with cooking spray and heat until medium-hot. Add the banana batter and cook for 2 to 3 minutes on each side. Serve topped with the berry applesauce.

375 calories, 10g fat, 60g carbs, 15g protein, 32g sugar

SERVES 1

Vegan French Toast

INGREDIENTS

- ½ cup unsweetened almond milk
- 1 teaspoon ground cinnamon
- ¼ cup fresh orange juice
- 1 teaspoon vanilla extract
- 2 slices Ezekiel or other sprouted grain bread
- Cooking spray
- Assorted toppings: agave, maple syrup, fresh berries

DIRECTIONS

In a medium bowl, whisk together the almond milk, cinnamon, orange juice, and vanilla. Dip the slices of bread in the liquid and let them sit in the mixture until it is absorbed.

Spray a skillet or griddle with cooking spray and place over medium-high heat. When hot, cook the bread slices for 2 or 3 minutes on each side, or until lightly browned. Top with toppings of your choice.

227 calories, 2g fat, 41g carbs, 9g protein, 9g sugar

SERVES 1

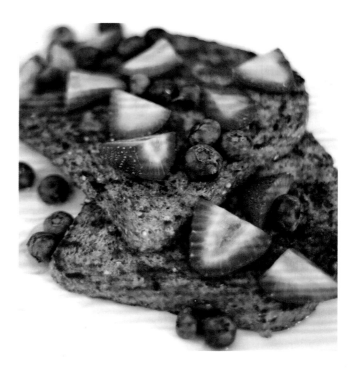

Flourless Pizza with Figs and Rosemary

INGREDIENTS

CRUST

- 1 cup shredded cauliflower florets
- ½ cup shredded mozzarella cheese
- 1 large egg
- 1 teaspoon dried oregano
- ½ teaspoon crushed garlic
- Cooking spray

TOPPING

- ⅓ cup nonfat cottage cheese
- 1 tablespoon balsamic vinegar
- 3 fresh figs, sliced
- 1 teaspoon chopped fresh or dried rosemary
- ½ cup chopped arugula

DIRECTIONS

Preheat the oven to 350°F.

Make the crust: Place the cauliflower in a microwave-safe bowl and cook on high for 8 minutes or until soft, almost a puree. Mix in the cheese, then crack the egg over it and mix in well with the oregano and garlic.

Coat a pizza pan with cooking spray and add the cauliflower puree, spreading it to make a nice base of "crust." Bake for 10 to 15 minutes, or until the crust is firm and lightly browned. Remove the crust but leave the oven on.

Make the topping: Place the cottage cheese in a blender and process until smooth. Spread it on the crust and drizzle with the vinegar. Top with the figs and sprinkle on the rosemary. Place the pizza back in the oven for another 10 minutes.

Top the pizza with the arugula and serve.

547 calories, 24g fat, 40g carbs, 45g protein, 27g sugar

SERVES 2

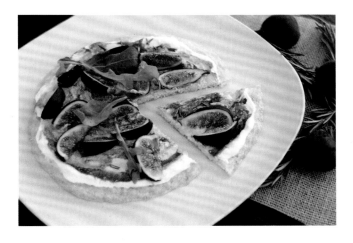

Egg(less) Salad Sandwich

INGREDIENTS

¾ cup cubed soft tofu

2 tablespoons vegan mayonnaise

2 teaspoons Dijon mustard

1 tablespoon chopped flat-leaf parsley

1 tablespoon chopped chives

Salt and pepper

2 slices Ezekiel or other sprouted grain bread

½ cup mixed baby greens

DIRECTIONS

Place the tofu in a mixing bowl and break it up with a fork. Mix in the mayonnaise, mustard, parsley, chives, and salt and pepper to taste. Cover and chill for about 30 minutes.

Assemble the sandwich by spreading the tofu mixture on the bread slices and top with the baby greens.

358 calories, 13g fat, 39g carbs, 21g protein, 3g sugar

SERVES 1

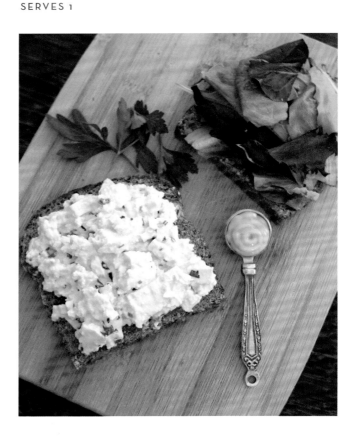

Summer Salad with Avocado Dressing

INGREDIENTS

SALAD

- 1 (4-ounce) cooked chicken cutlet, cut into cubes
- 1 cup chopped arugula
- 1 cup chopped fresh spinach
- 1 radish, thinly sliced
- ½ red bell pepper, seeded and sliced
- ½ cup chopped broccoli florets
- Dash of cracked black peppercorns

AVOCADO DRESSING

- ¼ ripe avocado
- ¼ cup chopped fresh cilantro
- ½ garlic clove, smashed
- 1 tablespoon lime juice
- Pinch of salt
- 1–2 tablespoons water, as needed

DIRECTIONS

Make the salad: In a bowl, combine and toss the salad ingredients.

Make the dressing: Combine the ingredients in a blender and process until smooth, using as much water as necessary to get the desired consistency.

Pour the dressing over the salad and toss.

238 calories, 11g fat, 11g carbs, 29g protein, 3g sugar

SERVES 1

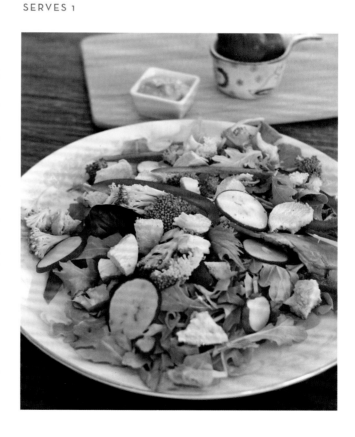

Eggplant Enchilada Tower with Zucchini Salsa Verde

INGREDIENTS

SALSA

- 2 teaspoons coconut oil
- 3 ¼-inch-thick slices Italian eggplant
- ½ medium zucchini, cut into chunks
- 1 tablespoon fresh lime juice
- ½ small jalapeño, seeded and trimmed
- ½ garlic clove
- ⅛ teaspoon ground cumin
- 1 teaspoon agave nectar

- 1 (4-ounce) chicken cutlet, cooked, cooled, and shredded
- 2 tablespoons plain 2% Greek yogurt

DIRECTIONS

Preheat the oven to 375°F.

Make the salsa: Place the coconut oil in a large skillet and heat on medium-high. Add the eggplant slices and sauté for 4 minutes on each side, until lightly browned.

Combine the zucchini, lime juice, jalapeño, garlic, cumin, and agave nectar in a blender. Process until smooth.

Add the salsa to the chicken in a bowl and mix to coat the chicken pieces.

Spray a baking sheet with cooking spray and place one eggplant slice on it and layer it with some of the chicken. Put another slice on top and layer it with more chicken. Add the remaining slice and the remaining chicken. Pat the sides and top to firm up the tower.

Bake for 15 minutes, or until warmed through. Top with the yogurt.

225 calories, 4g fat, 19g carbs, 30g protein, 9g sugar

SERVES 1

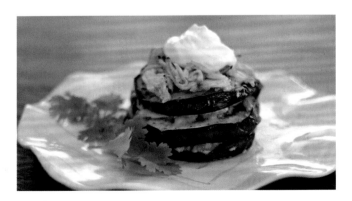

Cheesecake with Balsamic Berries

INGREDIENTS

BALSAMIC BERRY TOPPING

- 2 cups fresh berries of choice
- ¼ cup balsamic vinegar
- 1 teaspoon lemon zest
- 2 teaspoons stevia

CRUST

- 2 cups raw walnuts
- ½ cup dates, pitted

FILLING

- 3 cups raw cashews (soaked overnight or at least a couple of hours)
- ½ cup agave nectar
- ¼ cup lemon juice
- 1 teaspoon vanilla extract
- ¾ cup melted coconut oil (set in a warm bowl—do not heat if keeping this really *raw*)

DIRECTIONS

Make the berry topping: Place the berries in a bowl and add the vinegar, lemon zest, and stevia and toss carefully. Cover with plastic wrap and place in the refrigerator.

Make the crust: Place the walnuts and dates in a food processor and process until well combined. Press the mixture into an 8-inch pie pan.

Make the filling: Place all the filling ingredients in a food processor and process until smooth. Pour the filling into the pie crust and freeze for 3 hours.

When ready to serve, cut the cheesecake into eight slices and top each slice with some of the berry topping.

(for 1 slice): 225 calories, 4g fat, 19g carbs, 30g protein, 9g sugar

SERVES 8

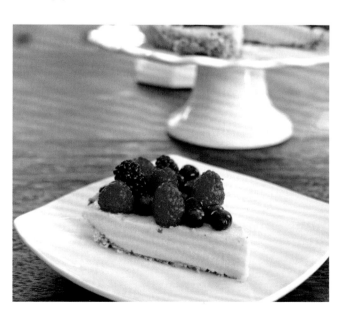

Peaches and Cream Pops

INGREDIENTS

1½ cups diced fresh peaches

1½ cups 2% vanilla Greek yogurt

DIRECTIONS

Place the peaches in a blender and blend until smooth. Pour the puree into a bowl and lightly stir in the yogurt.

Pour the mixture into ice pop molds and freeze overnight.

(for 1 pop): 67 calories, .2g fat, 10g carbs, 8g protein, 9g sugar

MAKES 8

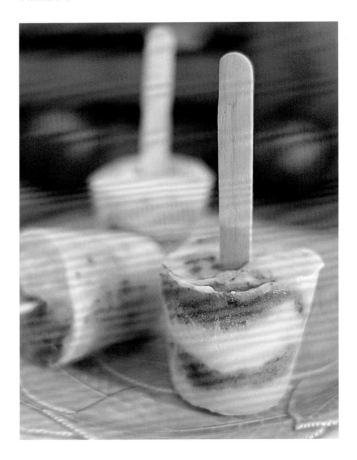

Fresh Fruit Salsa with Pita Chips

INGREDIENTS

SALSA

5 ripe strawberries, diced

1 mango, flesh diced

1 Persian cucumber, diced

1 small jalapeño, seeded and minced

1 tablespoon fresh lime juice

1 tablespoon chopped fresh mint

CHIPS

2 Ezekiel tortillas, cut into eighths

Olive oil spray

DIRECTIONS

Make the salsa: In a bowl, combine the salsa ingredients and lightly toss. Cover and chill.

Make the chips: Preheat the oven to 350°F. Lightly spray both sides of the tortilla slices with olive oil spray. Place on a baking sheet in a single layer and bake for 7 minutes. Flip over the slices and bake for another 7 minutes, until crisp and golden brown. Take out and let cool, then serve with the salsa.

(for the salsa): 89 calories, .6g fat, 26g carbs, 1g protein, 17g sugar

(for 8 chips): 150 calories, 4g fat, 24g carbs, 6g protein, 0g sugar

SERVES 2

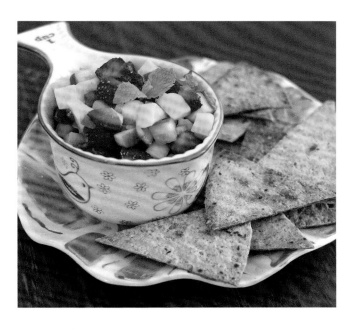

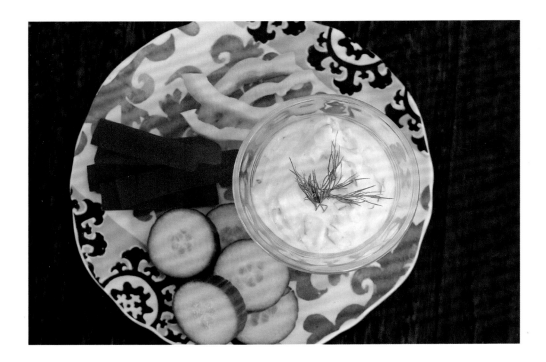

Veggies with Ranch Dip

INGREDIENTS

DRESSING

- ½ cup 2% plain Greek yogurt
- 1 tablespoon finely chopped fresh parsley
- 2 teaspoons finely chopped chives
- 1 teaspoon finely chopped fresh dill
- ½ garlic clove, minced

- 1 cup chopped seasonal veggies

DIRECTIONS

Make the dressing: Mix all the dressing ingredients in a bowl.

Serve with your favorite summer veggies.

(for the dressing): 80 calories, 0g fat, 6g carbs, 15g protein, 6g sugar

SERVES 1

A Note from Cassey

Why Confidence Is the Sexiest Thing a Woman Can Wear

Assessing physical beauty is so subjective. Rarely do you ever get a panel of judges to unanimously agree on the most attractive contestant in a pageant. But do you know what can't be denied? **True beauty that glows from the inside**—beauty that comes from a place of confidence, kindness, and health. You know a lovely woman when her smile makes you feel good about yourself.

You don't need a perfect hourglass figure or high cheekbones to be considered stunning. You just have to know that it doesn't matter what anyone else thinks. It only matters that you know **you're amazing.**

I once met a woman who walked in to a cocktail party wearing an old polo shirt tucked into her belted khakis. No makeup. Frizzy hair. All the other women were in high heels and tight dresses. I made a point of talking to her. Once she opened her mouth and started sharing her entrepreneurial adventures, her infectious drive and creativity took my breath away.

Confidence is the sexiest thing a woman can wear, in any season, regardless of the fashion. So, walk that sidewalk like it's your runway! Own everything you say, do, and teach! Home in on your talents, let them shine, and work the room like you mean it! You are one beautiful inspiration.

♡ Cassey

Summer Fast-Track Meal Plan

SUNDAY	MONDAY	TUESDAY	WEDNESDAY
Breakfast Pancakes with Berry Applesauce (page 133)	**Breakfast** Veggie scramble: 4 egg whites scrambled with 1 cup mixed veggies	**Breakfast** Vegan French Toast (page 134)	**Breakfast** High-fiber cereal with unsweetened almond milk and 2 tablespoons ground flaxseed
Snack ½ cup cottage cheese, 1 cubed nectarine	**Snack** 1 small banana, 1 tablespoon almond butter	**Snack** 15 almonds	**Snack** Fresh Fruit Salsa with Pita Chips (page 141)
Lunch Lunch salad: 4 cups mixed veggies/greens, 1 (4-ounce) cubed cooked chicken cutlet, and vinaigrette made with 1 tablespoon balsamic vinegar, 1 teaspoon olive oil, ½ tablespoon Dijon mustard	**Lunch** Summer Salad with Avocado Dressing (page 137)	**Lunch** Strawberry fields salad: 2 cups baby spinach, ⅓ cup sliced fresh strawberries, 8 walnuts, and 1 sliced nectarine, dressed with 2 teaspoons apple cider vinegar, 1 teaspoon olive oil, and 1 teaspoon honey	**Lunch** Egg(less) Salad Sandwich (page 136)
Snack 10 baby carrots, ¼ cup hummus	**Snack** 1 low-fat string cheese	**Snack** Veggies with Ranch Dip (page 142)	**Snack** 1 small banana, 1 tablespoon almond butter
Dinner Eggplant Enchilada Tower with Zucchini Salsa Verde (page 138)	**Dinner** Mediterranean quinoa: ½ cup cooked quinoa mixed with 1 small roasted beet, 1 Persian cucumber, 1 ounce crumbled feta, 1 tablespoon basil, 1 tablespoon balsamic vinegar	**Dinner** Flourless Pizza with Figs and Rosemary (page 135)	**Dinner** Leftover Flourless Pizza with Figs and Rosemary (page 135)

Recipes with page references are included in this book; others are quick and easy to put together in a flash!

THURSDAY	FRIDAY	SATURDAY
Breakfast 4 egg whites, 2 tomato slices, 1 slice whole wheat toast	**Breakfast** High-fiber cereal with unsweetened almond milk and 2 tablespoons ground flaxseed	**Breakfast** 2 scrambled egg whites, 2 ounces low-sodium turkey slices, 1 ounce mozzarella, 1 whole wheat English muffin
Snack Fresh Fruit Salsa with Pita Chips (page 141)	**Snack** ½ avocado, 1 teaspoon lemon juice	**Snack** ¾ cup mixed berries, 10 almonds
Lunch Quinoa bowl: ½ cup cooked quinoa, ¼ cup canned black beans, ½ cup chopped red bell pepper, 2 cups chopped fresh spinach	**Lunch** Chicken salad: 1 (4-ounce) cubed cooked chicken cutlet, 2 tablespoons plain 2% Greek yogurt, ½ diced apple, ½ teaspoon curry powder, served open-face on 1 slice of toast with ½ diced avocado sprinkled on top	**Lunch** Quinoa bowl: ½ cup cooked quinoa, 1 (4-ounce) diced cooked chicken cutlet, 2 cups chopped mixed greens, ¼ cup corn, 1 chopped tomato
Snack Plain 2% Greek yogurt (7-ounce container): eat plain or drizzle with 1 teaspoon of agave nectar	**Snack** 1 peach or nectarine	**Snack** Veggies with Ranch Dip (page 142)
Dinner Chicken and crunchy green beans: 1 (4-ounce) cooked chicken cutlet and 3 ounces sautéed green beans topped with 10 chopped almonds	**Dinner** Summer tofu sauté: Tofu cubes sautéed with 2 cups chopped summer veggies, 1 tablespoon soy sauce, and 1 teaspoon Sriracha hot sauce, served with ¼ cup cooked quinoa	**Dinner** Tacos: 3 ounces lean ground beef sautéed with ½ minced garlic, a pinch each of ground cumin and chili powder; wrap in a leaf of butter lettuce and top with 2% Greek yogurt and assorted chopped cooked veggies

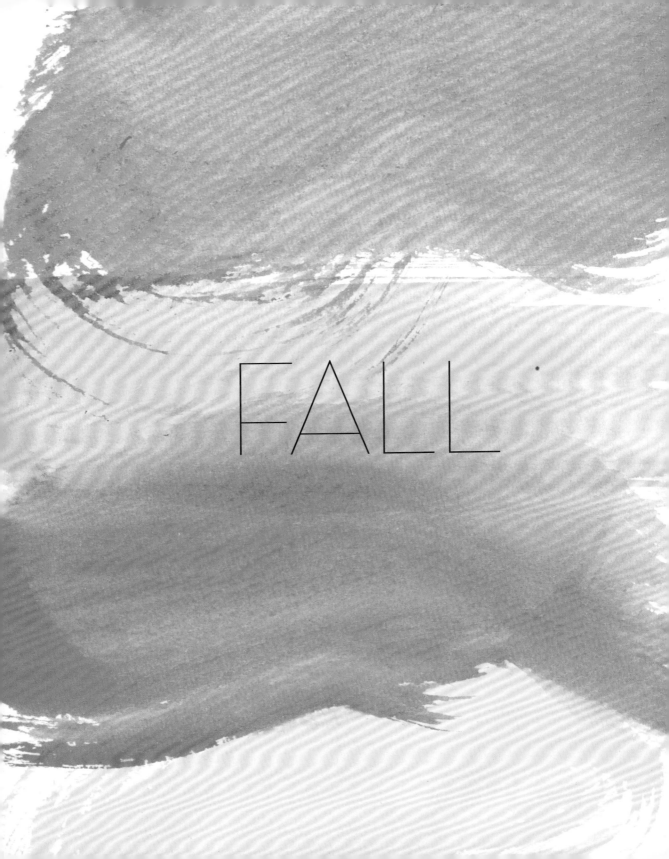

FALL

Fall

refocus, and stay active in changing weather

My favorite things about fall are its changing foliage and the smell of pumpkin and cinnamon. Don't you love them both? There's the coziness of wrapping yourself up in chunky sweaters and scarves, the thrill of seeing multi-hued leaves on the trees as you walk down the street. Yet at the same time you're getting back into the school routine. You have stacks of homework, the stress of tests, and even the simple task of learning a new subject. All that can really throw you into a whirlwind, especially if you're also trying to keep focus on your healthy eating and regular workouts.

If you're out of school and working now, you'll notice that the cooler weather may keep you inside longer. But don't succumb to that temptation! It's not yet winter, and there's no need to be trapped inside your office and then inside your home. Brisk neighborhood walks after dinner are refreshing, especially when you use them to zone out after a taxing day. Getting outside and moving will make you happy. Bring a friend along to make it an after-dinner date!

FALL MOVES

One of the most wonderful things about exercise and eating right is that both help your brain function and concentration. You'll be able to think sharper with a quick morning workout and a filling breakfast! You'll also have loads more energy for the day because you will have revved the engine of your metabolism.

Our sun-kissed summer memories are behind us now, but that doesn't mean we forget all the hard work we did to achieve that bikini body! With this new change of weather comes other changes: your skin gets chapped, you might start to feel emotionally low. There's a name for this condition: seasonal affective disorder, or SAD. Based on the shortened day length, the change of the season affects your mood, energy, and motivation. Honor those feelings but don't let them overcome you! Push that aside. Take advantage of the slight chill outside to fire up your own warmth from within.

LET'S GET FIERCE THIS FALL!

WORKOUT #1: TOTAL WAIST SLIMMING

Candlestick Dipper is my favorite muffin-top killer. It'll work your waist to shave off those pumpkin spice lattes.

CANDLESTICK DIPPER X 15 EACH SIDE
WORKS: OBLIQUES

A Start out on both knees, then extend your left leg straight out to the side, foot flat on the mat, toes forward. Bring your hands together, then raise your arms above your head. Beginners, bring your arms out to the sides, outstretched like airplane wings.

B Inhale and stretch your oblique to the right, away from your extended leg, and try to get your body parallel to the mat before going back up to start. Exhale on your way up. Keep your chest forward and your hips forward.

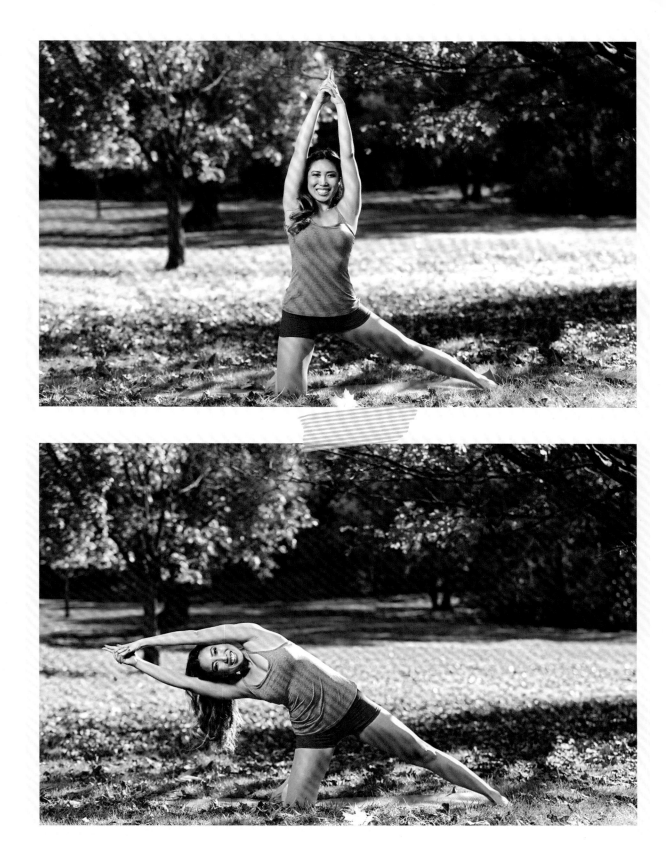

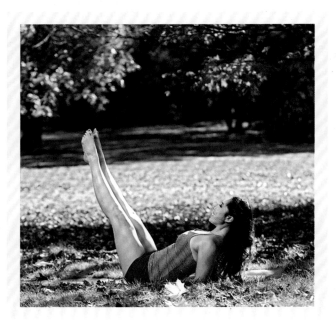

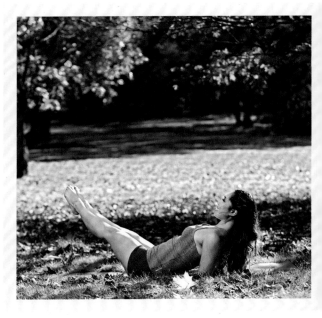

TRIANGLE CORKSCREW X 6 CLOCKWISE, 6 COUNTERCLOCKWISE
WORKS: LOWER ABS, QUADS

A Sit down and lean back as if you're basking in the sun, and prop yourself up on your elbows. Then lengthen your legs straight out to a diagonal as you balance on your tailbone and elbows.

B Draw a triangle with your toes, keeping your legs together and straight.

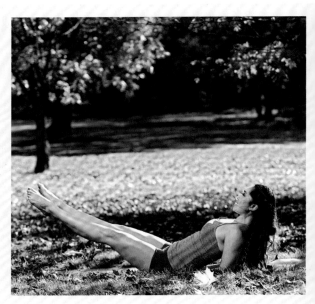

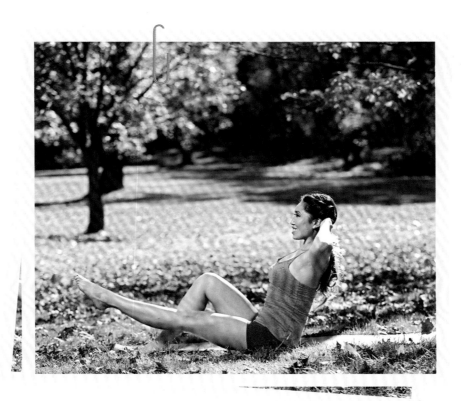

SINGLE-LEGGED SIT-UP
X 12 EACH LEG
WORKS: ABS, QUADS

A Lie down on your back and bring both of your hands behind the nape of your neck, keeping your elbows wide. Raise your left leg a few inches off the ground and hold it strong and straight.

B Exhale and do a full sit-up while keeping that leg stable and lifted off the mat. Inhale and roll down softly.

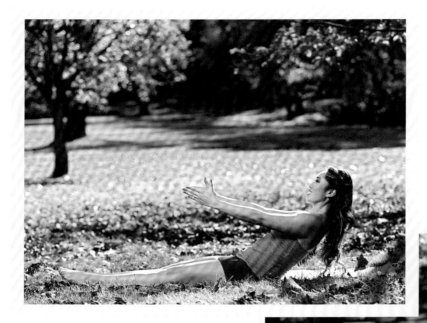

ALTERNATING EARTHQUAKE ELBOW TAP X 20 TAPS
WORKS: OBLIQUES, CORE

A Sit comfortably with your legs long, heels pressed together, toes pointed. Your back should be tall and your arms should be stretched forward. Lean back to your "tipping point," right before you're about to fall backward and you're just holding on with the strength of your core. Beginners, you may bend your knees and slightly curl your lower back to create a Pilates C-Curve.

B Twist and press your left elbow to the mat. Then alternate, pressing your right elbow to the mat.

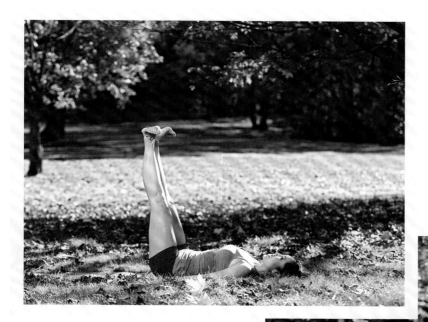

HEEL CLICK LEG LIFT X 12
WORKS: LOWER ABS, INNER THIGHS

A Lie on your back, head resting on the mat, and bring your hands into a triangle shape and place them right underneath your tailbone, your lower back pressed into the mat. Raise your legs straight up to the sky and flex your feet, heels together.

B Inhale and click your heels 4 times as you lower them to almost parallel to the mat, then exhale as you click 4 times to go up to the starting position. That counts as 1 leg lift. Do 12!

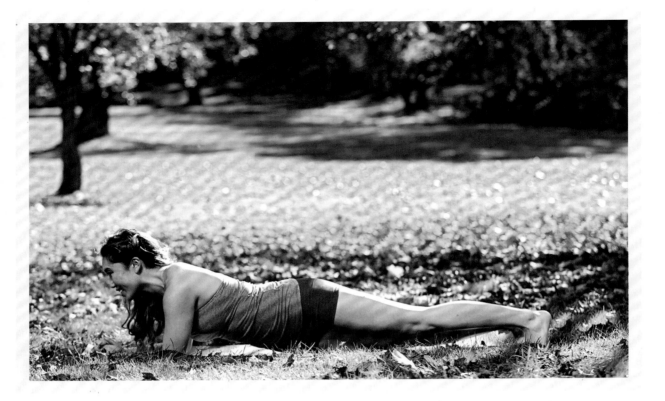

HIP TWISTING BUTT-UP
X 12
WORKS: OBLIQUES, SHOULDERS

A Get into Plank position on your elbows and toes. Your butt should be in line with the rest of your body—do not let the hips sink!

B Twist your right hip to touch the mat, twist your left hip to touch the mat, then flatten your back and raise your butt into the sky, and return to Plank.

Can't Stop Snacking?

The next time you find yourself snacking, think about what you were doing right before you went to the fridge to eat. Oftentimes, you are not hungry and you simply eat when you are bored or are trying to get away from doing something you don't like! Try grabbing a glass of water.

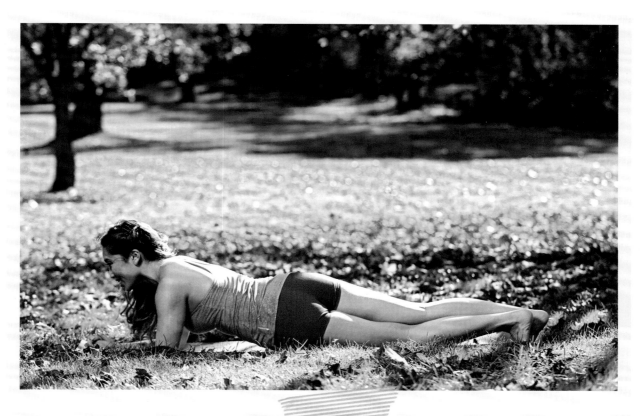

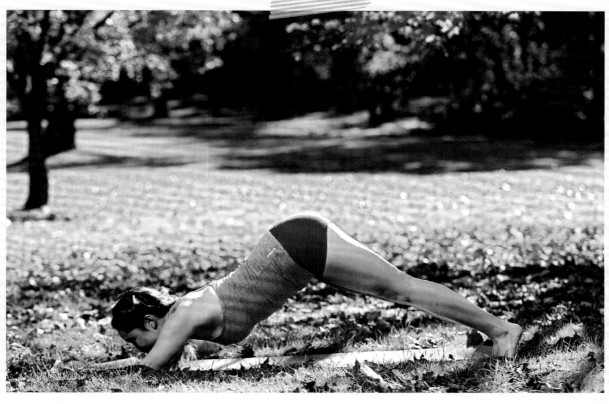

WORKOUT #2: AUTUMN BOTTOM

To tone your whole butt, you need to work your hamstrings, so I like to make sure that they are always at their strongest, as with the Jackhammer Extension. Try them, then fantasize that you're in warm Hawaii by channeling your inner Hula Dancer, working your butt and obliques while swaying your hips side to side.

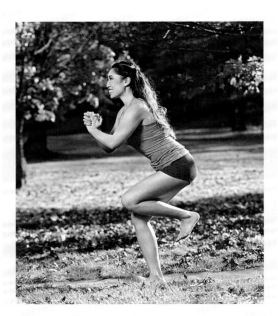 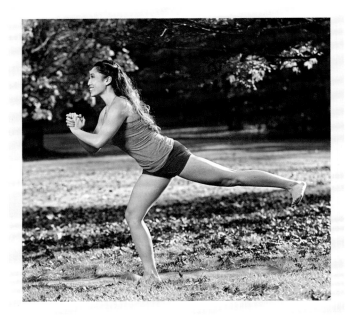

JACKHAMMER EXTENSION X 12 EACH LEG
WORKS: QUADS, GLUTEUS

A Begin with your right knee slightly bent into a Single-Legged Squat and your left foot flexed and off the mat. Your knees should be touching.

B Kick your left leg straight back, hold, and lift before returning to start. Keep the right knee in a slight squat at all times. Beginners, you may hold on to a wall or bar for better balance.

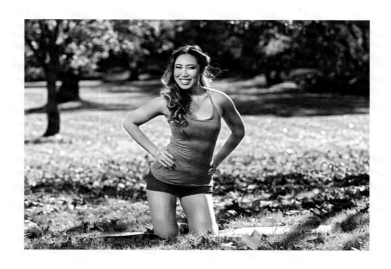

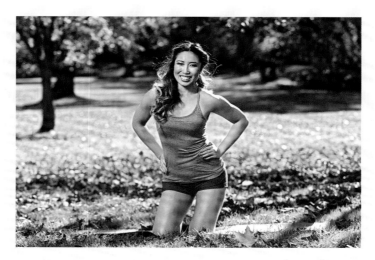

HULA DANCER X 40 SWAYS
WORKS: HIPS, QUADS

A You're on your knees with hands on your hips. Make sure your torso is tall.

B Sway your hips up to the left, then up to the right.

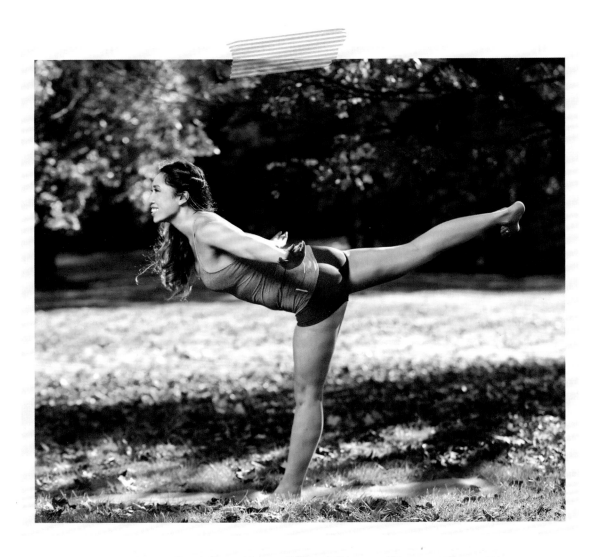

FLYING T-BUTT PULSE X 15 EACH LEG
WORKS: GLUTEUS, QUADS

A Balance on one leg and bring your chest forward with arms outstretched like a bird. Your back leg should be extended long behind you so that your body resembles a T.

B Lift and pulse your heel into the air, keeping both legs straight. When you lift, also squeeze your butt cheeks and hold for 1 second.

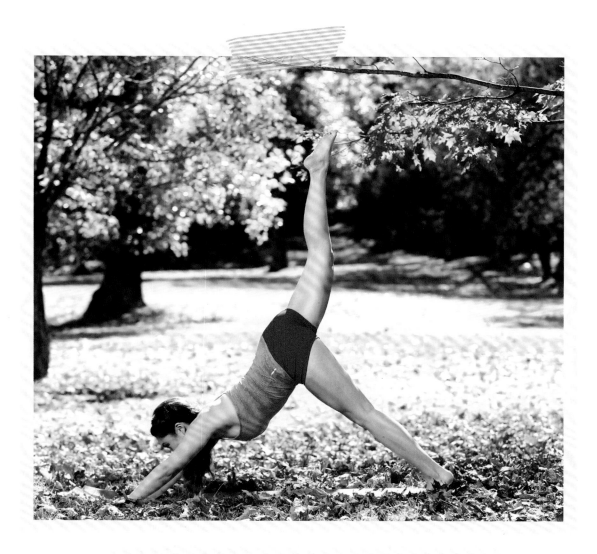

DOWN DOG LEG PULSE X 15 EACH LEG
WORKS: GLUTEUS, HAMSTRINGS

A Begin in a plank, your palms flat underneath your shoulders, belly button sucked in, tail bone tucked in, toes down. Draw your hips up into a Down Dog position.

B Then lift your right leg up into the air, hips square (meaning, don't open your hips to the side), point your toes, and pulse your leg up toward your back.

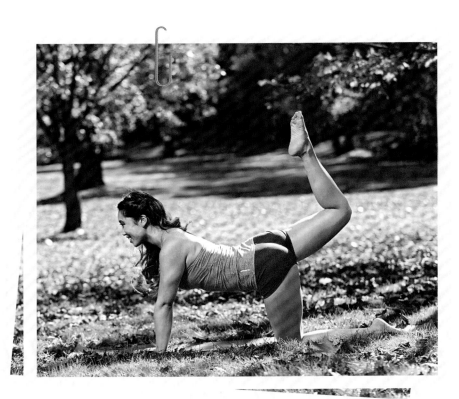

POINTED BUTT LIFT X 25 EACH SIDE
WORKS: GLUTEUS

A Begin on all fours, your hands underneath your shoulders, arms straight, knees about hip width apart. Lift your right leg up, knee bent at a 90-degree angle with your toes pointed into the air.

B Pulse and lift your leg up, hold, and squeeze your glutes before returning to the start position.

Stop Comparing Yourself

Comparison is the thief of joy. You are a different human being from the person standing next to you, and you have a different story and different goals. If you focus on making yourself stronger and better, and stop worrying about how your peers are doing, then you'll reach your fullest potential and achieve your goals much quicker. Trust in yourself! Believe.

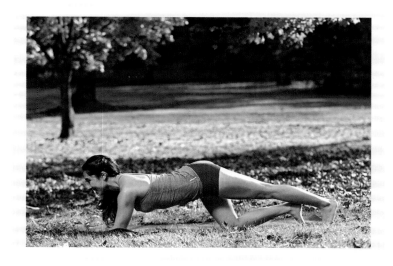

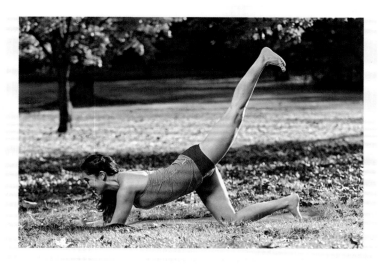

PRAYING HEEL LIFT X 20 EACH SIDE
WORKS: GLUTEUS, HAMSTRINGS

A Come down onto your forearms and knees. Then lift your left leg in the air, heel up, foot flexed.

B Bring your leg up and down, leading with the heel.

WORKOUT #3: LEGILATES

Wear your skinny jeans with heels this fall, because after this workout, your legs will be the stars of the show. Start with the Butterfly Squat to activate your calves and thighs, and end with the Standing Leg Circle for a big workout with an even bigger payoff.

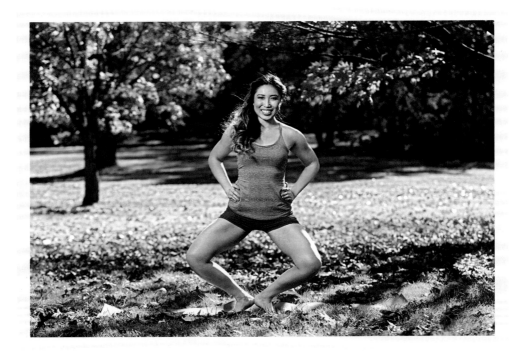

BUTTERFLY SQUAT X 10
WORKS: INNER THIGHS, OUTER THIGHS, CALVES

A Begin standing; place your hands on your hips and stand on the balls of your feet, feet at a diagonal, heels glued together and lifted.

B Press your knees out and in, and slowly lower yourself into a low squat with 4 butterfly wing flaps. Then slowly lift with 4 butterfly wing flaps up. This counts as 1 rep.

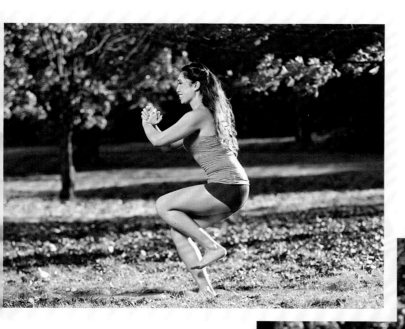

PEDAL PUSHER X 15 EACH LEG

WORKS: QUADS, GLUTEUS

A Begin in a low Single-Legged Squat with the right leg and bring your left knee up toward your chest, foot flexed.

B Exhale and press your left foot forward as if you're stepping on the gas. Inhale and bring it back to start, never getting up from the low Single-Legged Squat.

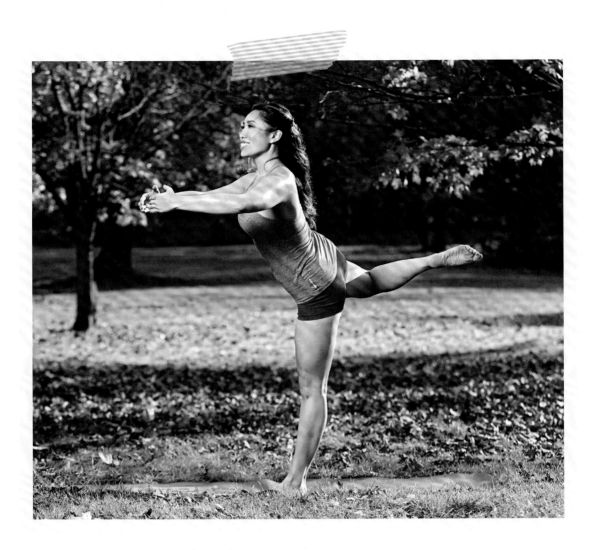

ATTITUDE PULSE X 15 EACH LEG
WORKS: GLUTEUS, THIGHS, LOWER BACK

A Stand on your left leg and lift your right knee behind you, opening up your inner thigh. Your arms should be in front of your body as if you're hugging a tree. Make sure your chin is up and your chest is open.

B Lift your knee up, then slightly lower it. This is one mini pulse.

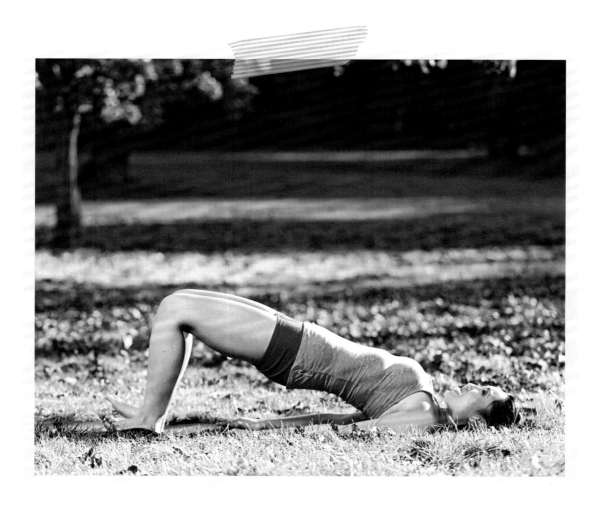

BRIDGE DIG THRUSTER X 25
WORKS: CALVES, HAMSTRINGS, GLUTEUS

A Lie on your back with arms resting by your side. Dig your heels into the mat, toes up, feet flexed, and lift your pelvis up into the air so that you're in Bridge position. The weight should be on your upper back and your heels.

B Lower your butt halfway to the mat and then exhale and press your pelvis as high as you can into the air. When you're up, squeeze your glutes as tight as possible. To make the move more advanced, move your heels farther from your body.

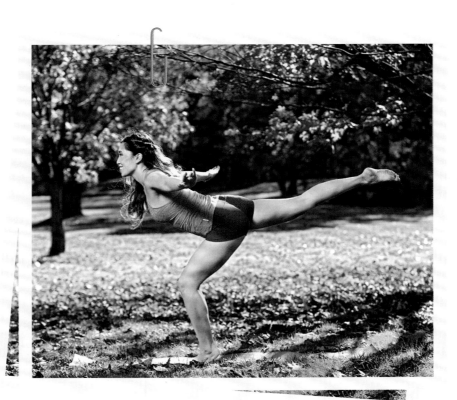

T-CALF RAISE X 12 EACH LEG
WORKS: CALVES, QUADS

A Begin in a standing T position with arms outstretched to the sides like a bird, with torso and lifted leg in one straight line, toes pointed. Lower yourself into a Single-Legged Squat with your standing leg's knee bent.

B Lift your heel up and lower it down, all while keeping your standing leg's knee bent.

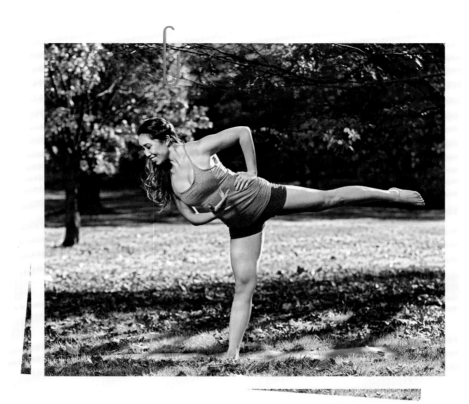

STANDING LEG CIRCLE X 10 FORWARD, 10 BACKWARD, EACH LEG

WORKS: GLUTEUS, INNER THIGHS, OUTER THIGHS

A Balance yourself on one leg and extend your other leg straight and long behind you. If you feel wobbly, you may hold on to a wall or chair.

B Keeping your core firm, allow your lifted leg to draw mini circles forward and backward.

Stressed?

Don't be. Worrying does nothing good for you. Instead, let go of that nervous energy by doing something you enjoy. For me, it's cooking, going to the farmer's market, taking a dance class, or working out—these activities can take my mind off any worrisome thoughts. The feel-good vibes that fill me after I do something I love are all the therapy I need to lower my stress.

WORKOUT #4: BACKLESS AND BEYOND

Go ahead! Go backless to your formal affair or work party; wear that favorite back-bearing dress once you've whipped that back into optimal shape with this workout. Hit your shoulders and arms with the Sky Reacher, then go Swimming to work your upper and lower back, and gain total body flexibility.

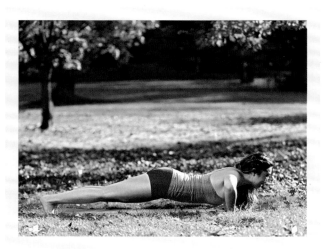 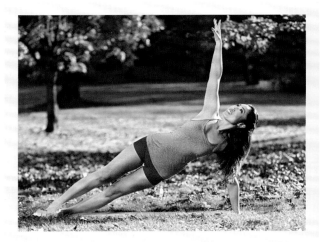

PUSH-UP TO SIDE PLANK X 12
WORKS: CHEST, ARMS, SHOULDERS

A Get into a push-up position on your toes and palms, or on your knees and palms if you're a beginner. Inhale, press your chest down to the mat as low as you can, then exhale pressing back up.

B Place your left hand below the center of your chest, open up your right arm, and come into a Side Plank with your feet stacked. Then return to start, do the push-up, and alternate your Side Plank.

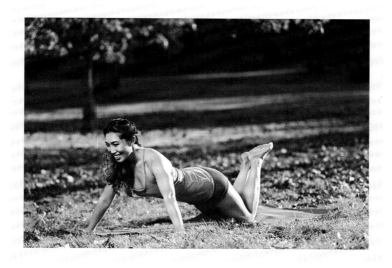

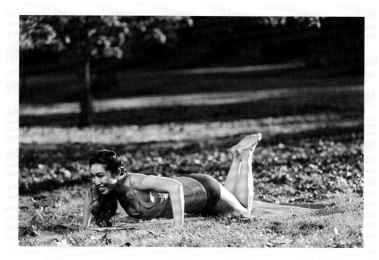

WIDE PUSH-UP TRIPLE PULSE X 12
WORKS: CHEST, ARMS

A On your knees, bring your arms outside the edge of your mat, in line with your shoulders. Your knees should be bent and your ankles crossed.

B Inhale and bring yourself down into a low push-up in beats of 3—3 presses down and 3 presses up. That's 1 rep.

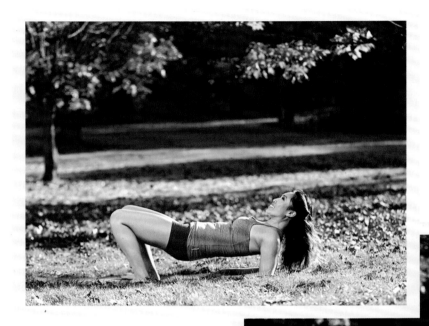

SKY REACHER X 20
WORKS: UPPER BACK

A Face your stomach to the sky and prop yourself up with your elbows. Your feet should be flat, hip width apart, pelvis up high.

B Reach your right arm toward the sky. Then switch and reach your left arm toward the sky.

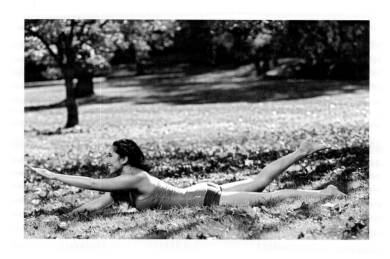

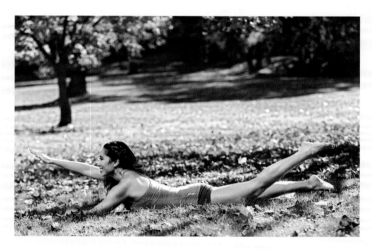

SWIMMING AT 30 SECONDS X 3
WORKS: UPPER BACK, LOWER BACK

A Lie on your stomach with your legs pointed behind you and your arms extended in front of you as if you're swimming. Lift your whole body up, chest off the mat, quads off the mat.

B Raise your left arm and your right leg, then raise your right arm and your left leg as quickly as possible, alternating for 30 seconds.

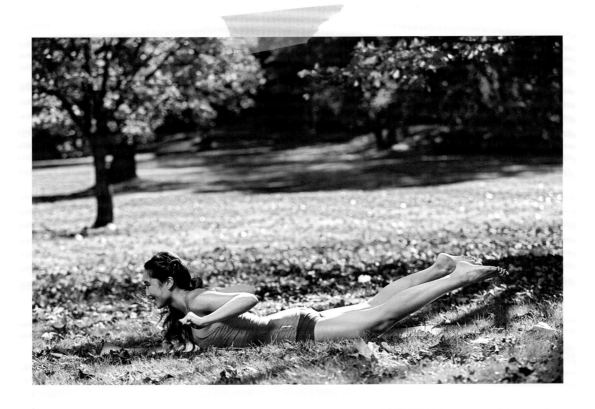

PARACHUTER X 20 NONSTOP

WORKS: UPPER BACK

A Lie on your stomach with your quads lifted off the mat, legs hip width apart, chest lifted, and elbows pressed back at a 90-degree angle.

B As you press your elbows into your mid-back, lift your chest higher and click your heels together. That's 1 rep.

Someone Said You Look "Fat"

This kind of comment can be such a hit to your self-esteem, but remember that a lot of times the person saying this is not comfortable in her own skin. Don't take it to heart; know that you are worth more than the number on the scale, and brush it off. We're all on our own fitness journeys, anyway.

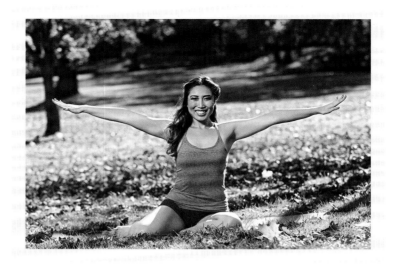

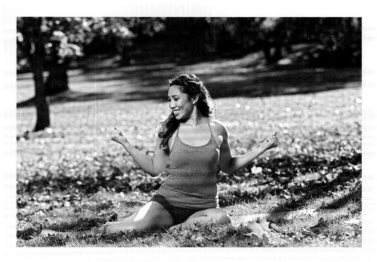

REACH 'N' PULL X 25
WORKS: SHOULDERS, MID-BACK

A Sit tall however you best feel comfortable. Stretch your arms long away from your body and to the sides, palms down.

B Exhale and pull your elbows behind your mid-back, as you clench your fists together, palms up, and tense your back and shoulders. Inhale and return to start.

WORKOUT #5: TOTAL BODY QUICK-FIX SLIM-DOWN

Time for your Total Body Slim-Down! Stay focused here and don't get discouraged—these moves are tough. Get yourself in game mode with the Reach Behind for core and balance, and rev up your heart rate with the Standing Roll-up. Then, my personal favorite, be stealthy with the Soldier Crawl—*get down and stay low!*

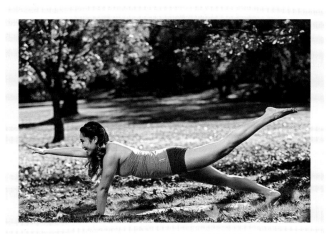 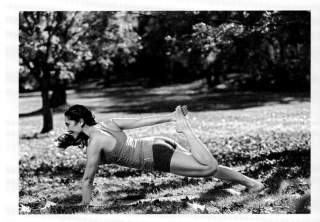

REACH BEHIND X 10
WORKS: CORE, CHEST, SHOULDERS

A Begin in Plank with hands underneath your chest, arms straight, and legs long behind you on your toes.

B Keeping your eyes forward and your hips square to the mat, lift your left leg and your right arm simultaneously and try to tap your toes with your fingers behind your back. Alternate sides. This is 1 rep.

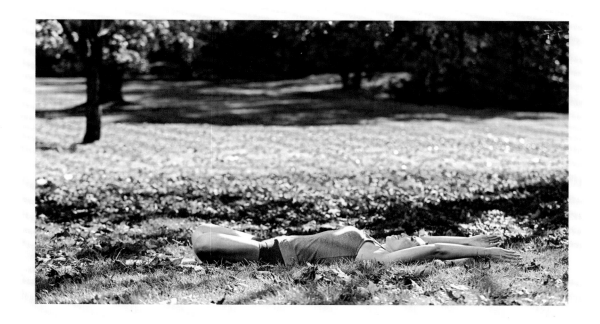

STANDING ROLL-UP X 12
WORKS: CARDIO, TOTAL LOWER BODY

A Begin with your legs crossed, lying down with your arms outstretched long behind you.

B Exhale and feel your spine get off the mat, bring your arms in front of you and stand up with your legs crossed, arms proudly in the air. Slowly lower yourself down and start again. Beginners, you can use your hands to assist and push you up as you stand up.

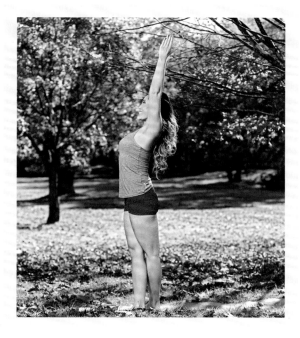

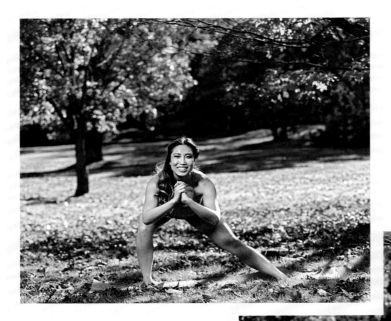

SIDE LUNGE TO TAP X 12 EACH SIDE
WORKS: INNER THIGHS

A Stand tall with your hands clasped in front of you. Bring your right leg out to the side and squat down with your left leg long and extended out to the side. Make sure your back is flat, your chest is high, and your butt is low.

B Keeping the left leg as straight as possible, press off of your right foot and bring it behind you, tapping your left fingers with your right toes. Repeat all reps on one side before moving on to the next.

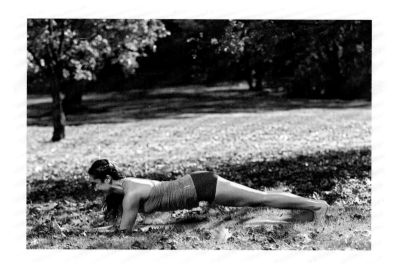

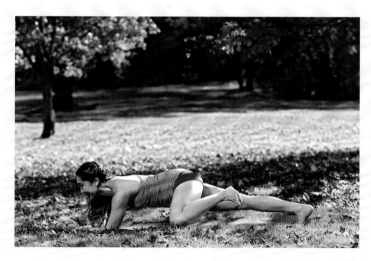

SOLDIER CRAWL X 20
WORKS: OBLIQUES, CORE

A Begin on your elbows in a Plank with your legs long behind you, balancing on your toes. Make sure your hips stay up. Beginners, you can perform Plank on your knees and elbows.

B Bring your left knee toward your elbow, hold, then press back to Plank. Alternate. This is 1 rep.

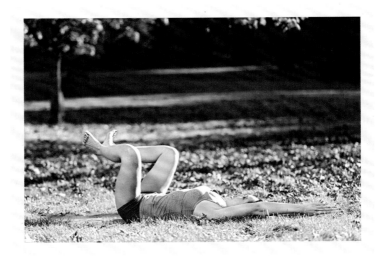

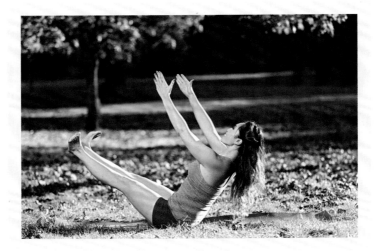

FROGGER ABS X 15
WORKS: INNER THIGHS, ABS

A Begin lying on your back with your arms long above your head. Your knees should be wide above your hips and your heels should be glued together, feet flexed.

B Exhale and press your heels forward while performing a sit-up. Bring your arms in front of you as your legs extend long, knees coming together. Inhale and roll slowly back to start.

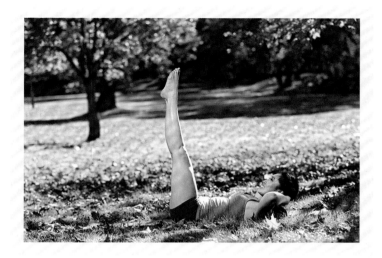

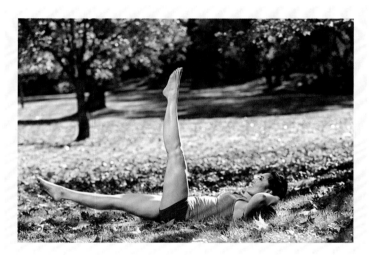

SINGLE-LEGGED DROP X 20
WORKS: LOWER ABS

A Place both hands behind the nape of your neck, elbows wide. Lift your upper body up into Pilates Stance, meaning, lift your head, neck, and shoulders up, eyes forward. Lift your legs up straight into the sky, feet pointed.

B Inhale and drop your right leg parallel to the floor, then exhale and lift it back up to meet your left leg. Then drop your left leg to the floor, exhale, and bring it back up. This is 1 rep.

A Note from Cassey

When No One Thinks You Can, and You Must

Have you ever felt so low because no one around you cares about your goals, your passions, and, well, you? I have. I've tried so hard to please other people and live their dreams instead of my own. I let myself become sculpted by their opinions of me and of my abilities. But you can only do this for so long. You break, and you never want to listen to anything these people say ever again.

When I say "break," I don't mean crumble. I mean you break those controlling opinions that mold you into someone you're not. But how do you do this?

What you need to do first is delete those people from your life. Get far, far away from them, because it's unhealthy for your mind and your spirit. Demeaning comments or condescending looks can seriously cripple your confidence. And I can't let that happen to you. Confidence is something that you need to caress and care for; it is the backbone of your existence!

If these people are your parents and you have to physically be around them, you'll need to block their opinions if they become damaging. You'll need to understand that you live for **you** and for anyone who cares about you wholeheartedly. Don't ever

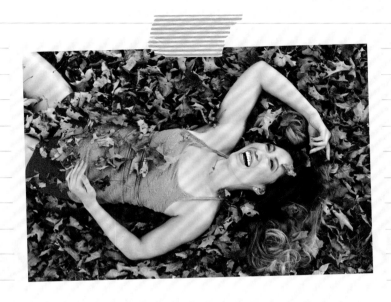

let anyone tamper with your hopes, your dreams, and your confidence ever again. In fact, use their doubts to fuel your passion. Think of it as a way to recycle the negative energy. I bet they'll be surprised.

I want you to know that you are capable of achieving everything you set your focus to achieve. If it's to lose weight, run faster, get admitted into the college of your dreams, or start your own business, there's nothing stopping you. It can be done and it has been done. All you have to do is write down your goal, keep it close to you, and look at it every day.

It only takes one person to ignite the process—you. So let's go. You deserve it.

♡ Cassey

FALL EATS

With the change in the leaves comes the change in available fruits and vegetables. Eating clean is really about embracing what the earth gives us, so in the fall I begin using root vegetables, cole crops, and winter squashes, and choosing the fall-ripening fruits like apples and pears. Instead of vibrant fruit salads, I transform ingredients to keep the heat in the kitchen, as in Cauliflower Chickpea "Couscous" (page 185). I pulse the cauliflower in a processor so that it looks and feels like a grain. And since the weather is a little colder, I use the oven for cooking dishes like Sunday's chicken plate, which roasts Brussels sprouts (yum!) in high heat—simultaneously making the house really cozy!

FALL'S IN-SEASON GROCERY LIST

Vegetables
acorn squash
arugula
Belgian endive
broccoli
Brussels
  sprouts
butter lettuce
butternut squash
cauliflower
daikon radish
endive
hot peppers
jicama
kale
pumpkin
radicchio
sweet potatoes
Swiss chard

Fruits
apples
Asian pears
cranberries
grapes
kumquats
pears
pomegranate

Mini Apple Crumble Protein Pancakes

INGREDIENTS

- ½ medium banana
- ¼ cup egg whites
- ½ apple, grated or cut into small matchsticks
- 2 tablespoons unsweetened vanilla almond milk or nonfat milk
- 1 teaspoon ground cinnamon
- ¼ teaspoon ground nutmeg
- 1 tablespoon ground flaxseed
- Cooking spray
- 1 tablespoon finely chopped walnuts (optional)

DIRECTIONS

In a large mixing bowl, mash the banana with the back of a spoon or a fork. Add the remaining ingredients except the walnuts, and stir until well combined.

Coat a nonstick skillet with cooking spray. Pour ¼ cup of the batter into the pan. Once it begins to bubble, 30 seconds to 1 minute, flip the pancake and cook for another 20 to 30 seconds. Repeat with the remaining batter.

Top with the walnuts, if desired, and serve.

(for 1 pancake): 272 calories, 12g fat, 29g carbs, 19g protein, 17g sugar

SERVES 1

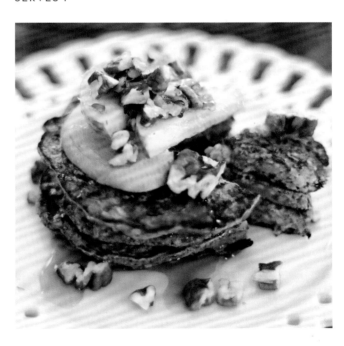

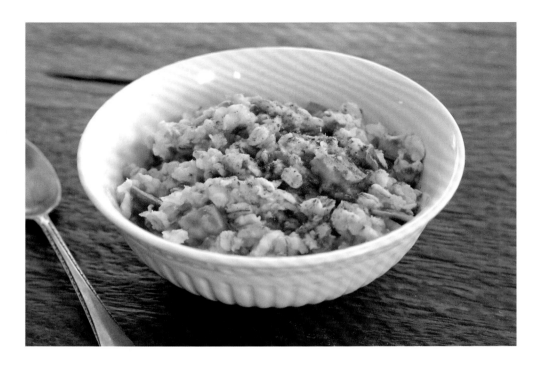

Sweet Potato Oatmeal

INGREDIENTS

- ⅓ medium sweet potato, peeled and cut into ½-inch cubes
- ¼ cup old-fashioned rolled oats
- ¾ to 1 cup unsweetened vanilla almond milk
- 1 tablespoon ground flaxseed
- 1 teaspoon ground cinnamon
- 1 tablespoon maple syrup

DIRECTIONS

In a small microwave-safe bowl, microwave the sweet potato on high for 3 to 4 minutes, or until soft. Roughly smash with the back of a spoon or a fork.

Place the oats, almond milk, flaxseed, and sweet potato in a medium saucepan. Bring almost to a boil, then reduce the heat to low, cover, and simmer for 10 minutes, until the oats are creamy.

Add the cinnamon and maple syrup, stir until combined, and serve.

288 calories, 6g fat, 51g carbs, 7g protein, 19g sugar

SERVES 1

Cauliflower Chickpea "Couscous"

INGREDIENTS

- 1 cup coarsely chopped cauliflower florets
- 1 teaspoon olive oil
- ⅓ cup diced zucchini
- 1 carrot, shredded
- ½ cup canned chickpeas (garbanzo beans), drained and rinsed
- ¼ teaspoon ground cumin
- ¼ teaspoon ground coriander
- ½ teaspoon shredded fresh ginger
- ⅓ cup low-sodium vegetable stock
- 1 tablespoon golden raisins
- 2 cups chopped fresh spinach

DIRECTIONS

Place the cauliflower in a food processor and pulse until it is the texture of rice.

Heat the olive oil in a medium nonstick skillet over medium-high heat and add the zucchini, carrot, chickpeas, cumin, coriander, and ginger. Sauté until the vegetables just begin to soften, about 3 minutes.

Add the stock and raisins. Reduce the heat and simmer for 3 minutes. Add the spinach and cauliflower, and cook until the spinach is wilted, about 2 minutes.

323 calories, 7g fat, 60g carbs, 11g protein, 17g sugar

SERVES 1

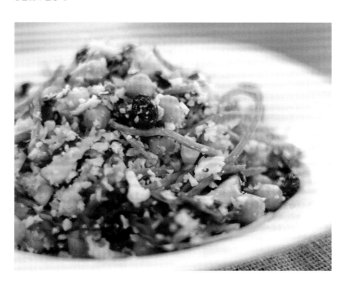

Turkey Quesadilla

INGREDIENTS

2 tablespoons cranberry sauce

1 tablespoon chopped fresh cilantro

1 sprouted grain 8-inch tortilla

2 tablespoons shredded mozzarella cheese

1 (4-ounce) turkey cutlet, cooked, cooled, and shredded

2 tablespoons 2% Greek yogurt

DIRECTIONS

In a small bowl, mix the cranberry sauce with the cilantro. Spread on the tortilla. Sprinkle the cheese on half of the tortilla. Top with the turkey.

Heat a medium nonstick skillet over medium heat. Fold the tortilla over the filling and place in the hot skillet. Cook for 3 minutes on each side, until lightly browned. Top with the yogurt.

345 calories, 10g fat, 36g carbs, 29g protein, 10g sugar

SERVES 1

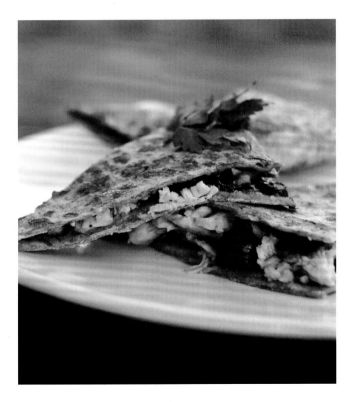

Chicken Alfredo with Zucchini Noodles

INGREDIENTS

CASHEW CREAM

8 raw cashews

¼ cup water

1 teaspoon olive oil

1 (4-ounce) chicken cutlet, cut into cubes

1 cup chopped broccoli florets

½ cup chicken stock

2 tablespoons grated Parmesan cheese

Pinch of freshly grated nutmeg

1 medium zucchini, sliced thinly with a mandoline, then steamed for 1 minute

2 tablespoons chopped fresh parsley

DIRECTIONS

Make the cashew cream: Soak cashews in water for 2 to 3 hours. Blend the cashews and water in a food processor until creamy.

Heat the oil in a large nonstick skillet over medium-high heat. Add the chicken and sauté 5 to 6 minutes, stirring occasionally, until cooked through. Remove from the skillet.

Add the broccoli to the skillet and sauté for 3 to 4 minutes, stirring occasionally, until tender. Add the stock and lower the heat to a simmer. Stir in the cashew cream, Parmesan, nutmeg, and chicken. Heat through.

Toss in the zucchini noodles and parsley, stir, and heat until warmed through.

334 calories, 16g fat, 15g carbs, 34g protein, 4g sugar

SERVES 1

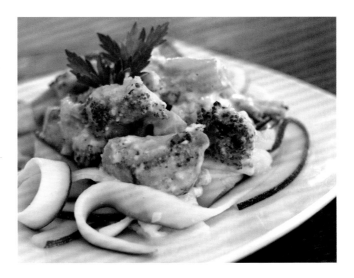

Curried Squash Stew

INGREDIENTS

- 1 teaspoon olive oil
- 2 tablespoons minced red onion
- 1 garlic clove, minced
- ½ teaspoon ground ginger
- ½ teaspoon curry powder
- ½ cup cubed (1-inch) peeled butternut squash
- ¼ cup light coconut milk
- 1 cup vegetable stock
- ¼ cup canned chickpeas (garbanzo beans), rinsed and drained
- ¼ red bell pepper, seeded and cut into 1-inch cubes
- 1 cup chopped fresh kale, thick stems removed
- 1 teaspoon fresh lemon juice
- Salt and pepper to taste
- 1 tablespoon chopped fresh cilantro

DIRECTIONS

Heat the oil in a large pot over medium heat. Sauté the onion and garlic for 2 minutes, stirring frequently. Stir in the ginger and curry powder, then add the squash and cook for 2 minutes.

Stir in the coconut milk and vegetable stock, and bring to a boil. Lower the heat and cover. Simmer for 10 minutes.

Add the chickpeas and red pepper. Cook for 5 minutes, or until the pepper and squash are cooked through.

Stir in the kale, lemon juice, and salt and pepper. Simmer for 2 to 3 minutes, until the kale is slightly wilted. Sprinkle with the cilantro and serve.

271 calories, 12g fat, 38g carbs, 8g protein, 5g sugar

SERVES 1

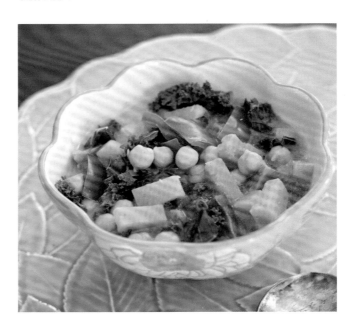

Banana Pecan Ice Cream Parfait

INGREDIENTS

- 1 teaspoon coconut oil
- 1 tablespoon roughly chopped pecans
- ½ tablespoon maple syrup or agave nectar
- 1 ripe banana, sliced and frozen

DIRECTIONS

Heat the oil in a small skillet over medium heat. Add the pecans and cook for 2 minutes, until lightly toasted. Stir in the maple syrup and heat through, then remove from the heat.

Blend the frozen banana slices in a blender for 2 to 3 minutes, scraping down the sides occasionally. Scoop into a bowl and top with the pecans.

268 calories, 15g fat, 35g carbs, 3g protein, 21g sugar

SERVES 1

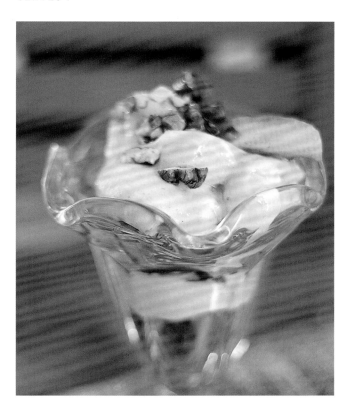

Baked Pear

INGREDIENTS

- 1 tablespoon maple syrup
- ½ teaspoon ground cinnamon
- ⅓ cup unsweetened vanilla almond milk
- 1 Bosc pear
- ½ cup banana ice cream (optional)

DIRECTIONS

Preheat the oven to 400°F.

In a medium bowl, whisk together the syrup, cinnamon, and almond milk. Pour three-fourths of the mixture into a small glass baking dish. Place the pear in the almond milk mixture, and spoon the rest of the mixture over the top.

Bake the pear for 40 minutes, basting with the almond milk mixture every 10 minutes, until softened. Serve à la mode with banana ice cream, if desired.

160 calories, 1g fat, 38g carbs, 1g protein, 28g sugar

SERVES 1

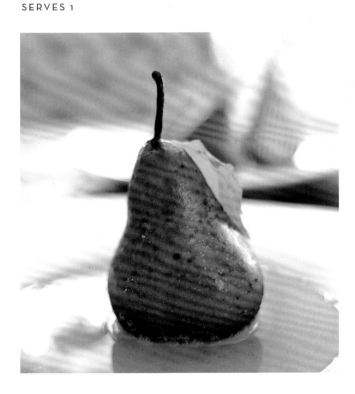

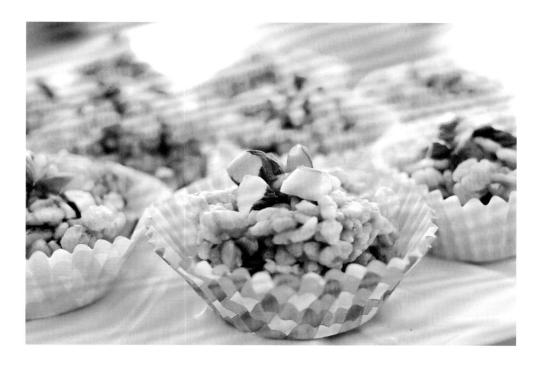

Crispy Rice Treat Energy Morsels

INGREDIENTS

⅓ cup reduced-fat peanut butter

⅓ cup agave nectar

2 cups brown rice cereal

¼ cup chopped almonds

¼ cup dried cranberries

DIRECTIONS

Line two full-size muffin tins with paper liners and set aside.

Heat the peanut butter and agave nectar in a large saucepan over low heat for about 5 minutes, stirring constantly, until smooth, melted, and bubbling just a bit.

Turn off the heat, add the cereal, almonds, and cranberries to the mixture and carefully stir until well combined.

Fill the muffin cups with the mixture and let cool.

(for 1 morsel): 113 calories, 5g fat, 16g carbs, 3g protein, 7g sugar

MAKES 10 MORSELS

Coconut Power Balls

INGREDIENTS

- 1 cup raw walnuts
- 5 pitted dates
- 1 tablespoon toasted shredded coconut

DIRECTIONS

Pulse the walnuts and dates in a food processor until well combined. Roll into 1-inch balls, using your hands. Coat with the coconut, and place in the refrigerator for at least 1 hour to firm up.

(for 1 ball): 170 calories, 15g fat, 10g carbs, 3.4g protein, 6g sugar

MAKES ABOUT 5 BALLS

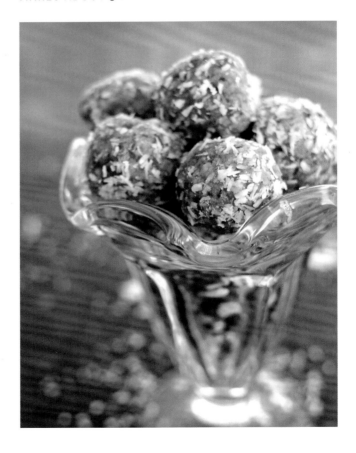

A Note from Cassey

Why Indulging Is Okay—Why You Shouldn't Feel Guilty

Don't let a stumble in the road bring you to a complete halt along your journey. You've got to get back up and keep going. The desire to keep moving forward regardless of the hardships you've endured is what builds character and true strength. This is what I call resilience.

So many times I've felt so hopeless and frustrated that, after a month of hard training and clean eating, a simple week of travel can completely set me back. Everything that I've worked for can be erased just like that? It's heartbreaking. It's depressing. It makes me want to just quit.

But I can't. I **can't** feel sorry for myself. I must continue. I must persevere!

There's no such thing as giving up on yourself! If you don't believe you can pick up the pieces and try again, know that no one else is going to do it for you. The experiences you've gained through your journey are yours to keep, so use them to get back up and running even quicker than when you started.

Still feeling down? No! A little weight gain, a little tiredness—that's nothing you can't fix because you've done this before. Let go of the past to make space for the new future. Show me your power! Show me your resilience.

Let's go!

♡ Cassey

Fall Fast-Track Meal Plan

SUNDAY	MONDAY	TUESDAY	WEDNESDAY
Breakfast Mini Apple Crumble Protein Pancakes (page 183)	**Breakfast** Mexican eggs: 4 scrambled egg whites, ⅓ cup salsa, 1 slice of toast, ¼ diced avocado	**Breakfast** Sweet Potato Oatmeal (page 184)	**Breakfast** High-fiber cereal with unsweetened almond milk and 2 tablespoons ground flaxseed
Snack 2 rice crackers with 1 low-fat string cheese	**Snack** Crispy Rice Treat Energy Morsels (page 191)	**Snack** Plain 2% Greek yogurt drizzled with 1 teaspoon agave (optional)	**Snack** 1 apple with 1 tablespoon peanut butter or almond butter
Lunch Cauliflower Chickpea "Couscous" (page 185)	**Lunch** Tuna sandwich: ½ can tuna (5 ounces) mixed with 2 teaspoons mustard, 2 chopped small pickles, and 1 tablespoon vegan mayo, on 2 slices sprouted grain bread and topped with mixed greens	**Lunch** Lunch salad: 4 cups mixed cooked veggies or lettuce and 1 (4-ounce) chopped cooked chicken cutlet tossed with vinaigrette of 1 tablespoon balsamic vinegar, 1 teaspoon olive oil, and ½ tablespoon Dijon mustard	**Lunch** Lettuce wraps: 2 large lettuce leaves filled with 1 (4-ounce) shredded cooked chicken cutlet and 1 cup assorted raw veggies (shredded carrots, Persian cucumber, tomato), with ¼ cup hummus split between the two wraps
Snack 1 cup steamed edamame	**Snack** 1 apple with 1 tablespoon peanut butter or almond butter	**Snack** Crispy Rice Treat Energy Morsels (page 191)	**Snack** 3 slices low-sodium turkey with 1 low-fat string cheese
Dinner Chicken plate: 1 cooked medium sweet potato, 1 (4-ounce) cooked chicken cutlet, and 1 cup roasted Brussels sprouts (cut in half, tossed with extra-virgin olive oil spray, and roasted at 400°F for 20 minutes)	**Dinner** Tofu and veggies: ⅓ cup cubed tofu sautéed with 2 teaspoons olive oil, 4 button mushrooms, ½ cup zucchini, ½ cup broccoli, 2 cups baby spinach, and 1 tablespoon lemon juice	**Dinner** Salmon plate: 1 (4-ounce) baked salmon fillet (350°F, 15 minutes) with 1 cup steamed broccoli tossed in 1 teaspoon extra-virgin olive oil and salt and pepper to taste	**Dinner** Curried Squash Stew (page 188)

Recipes with page references are included in this book; others are quick and easy to put together in a flash!

THURSDAY	FRIDAY	SATURDAY
Breakfast Protein smoothie: 1 scoop of protein powder, 1 cup chopped raw kale, 1 small frozen banana, ½ pear	**Breakfast** High-fiber cereal with unsweetened almond milk and 2 tablespoons ground flaxseed	**Breakfast** Banana oatmeal: 1 cup cooked oatmeal, 1 mashed small banana, and 1 teaspoon agave nectar
Snack Crispy Rice Treat Energy Morsels (page 191)	**Snack** ½ cup broccoli florets with ¼ cup hummus	**Snack** 1 cup steamed edamame
Lunch Turkey sandy: 4 ounces low-sodium turkey slices, 2 tomato slices, 1 cup mixed greens on whole wheat English muffin	**Lunch** Turkey Quesadilla (page 186)	**Lunch** Protein smoothie: 1 scoop of protein powder, 1 cup chopped raw kale, 1 small frozen banana, ½ pear
Snack 1 celery stalk and 1 carrot with ¼ cup hummus	**Snack** Crispy Rice Treat Energy Morsels (page 191)	**Snack** Plain 2% Greek yogurt with 1 teaspoon agave (optional)
Dinner Breakfast for dinner: 4 scrambled egg whites sprinkled with Parmesan cheese, 1 slice of Ezekiel (or sprouted grain) toast, and ¼ diced avocado	**Dinner** Dinner salad: 4 cups mixed raw veggies or lettuce and 1 (4-ounce) diced cooked chicken cutlet tossed with vinaigrette of 1 tablespoon lemon juice, 1 teaspoon olive oil, ½ tablespoon Dijon mustard, and 1 teaspoon agave nectar	**Dinner** Chicken Alfredo with Zucchini Noodles (page 187)

WINTER

Winter
chill out during the stress, manage the holiday activities without guilt

The holidays are upon us! I can hear the sound of wood crackling in the fireplace, see my neighbors' houses dancing with lights in the evening, feel everyone's laughter in the air, and taste the mouthwatering hors d'oeuvres at those holiday parties. This is the time when your family whips up the most indulgent meals of the year!

The battle to get up and work out during the winter is tough, and the struggle to eat clean foods is nearly torture. So this is what I suggest. Don't deprive yourself of these amazing foods, because eating is a part of the human experience. Instead, have a little of them and embrace the flavors of the season. You may also want to stick to the rule of one YOLO meal* a week, which will keep you sane. Try to fill yourself with lean proteins and veggies before you attend a holiday party so you won't fall prey to those pretty pastries.

Keep reminding yourself how good you felt in the spring and summer—lighter and cleaner—because then it truly was easy to step outside and prance in the sun, or to dig through the abundance of fresh fruits and veggies at the market. Although your plates might not be full of fruity colorful salads at this time of year, you can still be creative

....

*You Only Live Once meal is a meal in which you can eat whatever you want!

and whip up a veggie-packed stew, soup, or casserole to keep you warm and full of nutrients. Just because your clothes are heavy doesn't mean your food needs to be, too. Keep away from the heavy sauces, creams, and butters when working your magic in the kitchen, and find creative ways to flavor: use herbs such as sage, rosemary, and thyme! The options are limitless if you open your eyes and get excited about what you're preparing.

Remember: don't be too hard on yourself. The holidays come only once a year. Enjoy them! As long as you keep training passionately and eating nutritiously, you will be perfect.

STAY STRONG, BE RESILIENT, AND GOOD LUCK! LET'S CONQUER THIS WINTER WONDERLAND!

WINTER MOVES

WORKOUT #1: MUFFIN-TOP MELTDOWN

Leave the jolly belly to Santa this winter, and maintain a slim middle. You'll thank me when the weather warms up! Choreographed, multilayered moves like the Shooting Star are a fun and inspiring method for burning off those holiday sweets.

TRUNK TWIST X 20 TAPS
WORKS: OBLIQUES, QUADS

A Place your hands in front of you, your forearms creating a straight line from elbow to elbow. Balance on your tailbone with your legs lifted off the mat, ankles crossed, knees bent. Beginners, you may rest your feet on the mat.

B Inhale and twist as you tap your left elbow down to the mat, exhale up toward center, and inhale as you twist your right elbow down to tap.

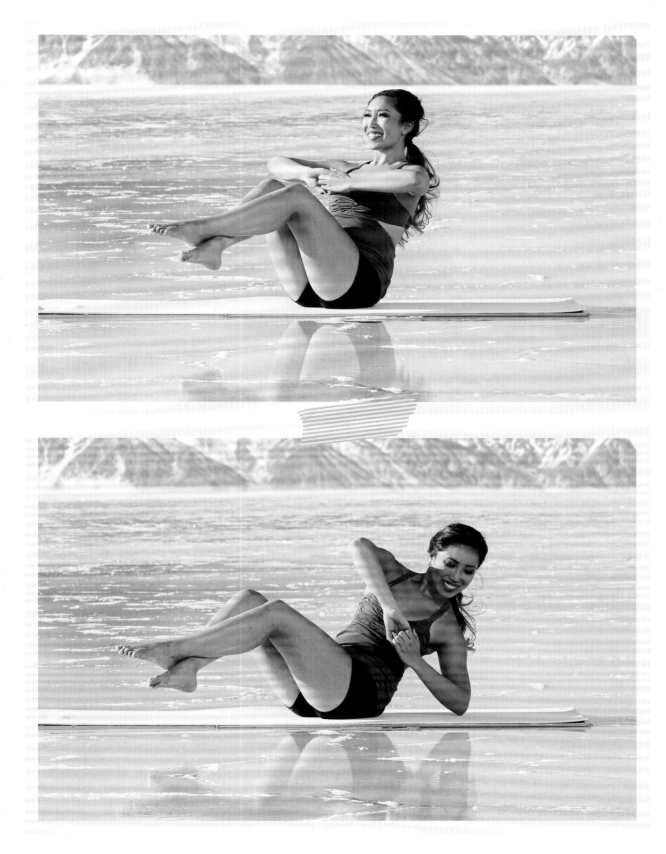

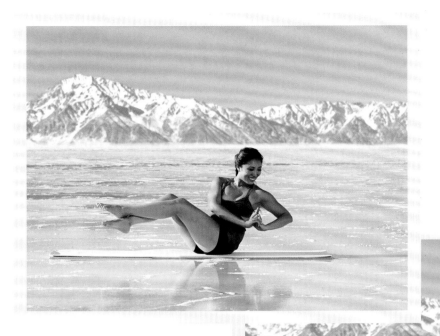

SHOOTING STAR X 15 SHOTS
WORKS: OBLIQUES, ABS, SHOULDERS, QUADS

A Place your hands in a Charlie's Angel position, hands held together with pointer fingers up like a gun. Your legs should be lifted off the mat, ankles crossed, knees bent with your torso sitting tall, balanced on your tailbone. Beginners, you may leave both feet on the mat.

B Inhale and tap the tip of your gun to the left side of your hip, exhale and extend your legs forward long and straight while bringing your gun above your head and shoot! Then inhale down to the right.

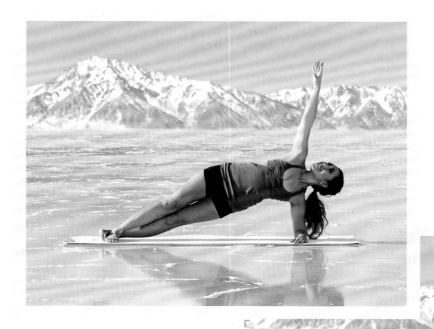

SIDE PLANK ROTATOR X 10 EACH SIDE
WORKS: OBLIQUES, SHOULDERS, CORE

A Balance yourself in a Side Plank on your left elbow and feet. Your elbow should be directly underneath your shoulder and your top leg should be crossed over your bottom at the ankle. Raise your right arm to the sky and keep your eyes on your fingers at all times.

B Exhale and curve your right hand underneath your belly. Inhale and lift your right arm back up again.

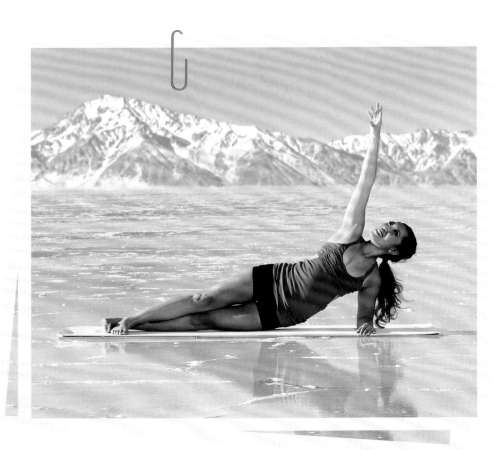

SIDE PLANK DIP X 10 EACH SIDE
WORKS: OBLIQUES

A Place your left elbow beneath your shoulder and prop yourself up into a Side Plank. Your legs should be long, top leg crossed over the bottom leg at the ankle. Raise your right arm to the sky and keep your eyes on your fingers.

B Keeping your hips and chest forward, tap your bottom hip to the mat, then lift back up into Side Plank. Beginners, you can perform this move on your elbow and knees.

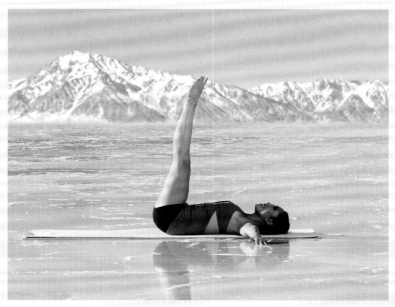

WINDMILL X 12
WORKS: OBLIQUES, LOWER BACK

A Lie flat on your back, head resting on the mat, arms out to the side, palms pressed into the ground. Lift both your legs straight up, heels pressed together, toes pointed.

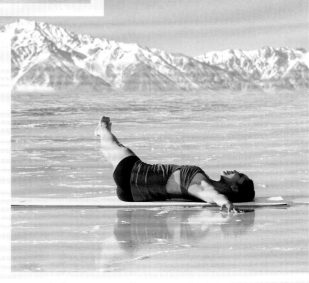

B Inhale and take the legs as one unit to the right side of your body as low as you can go without lifting your upper back off of the mat. Then exhale, bring your legs back to center, and inhale down to the left. That's 1 rep. Beginners, you may bend your knees at a 90-degree angle in Tabletop position as you windmill yourself from side to side.

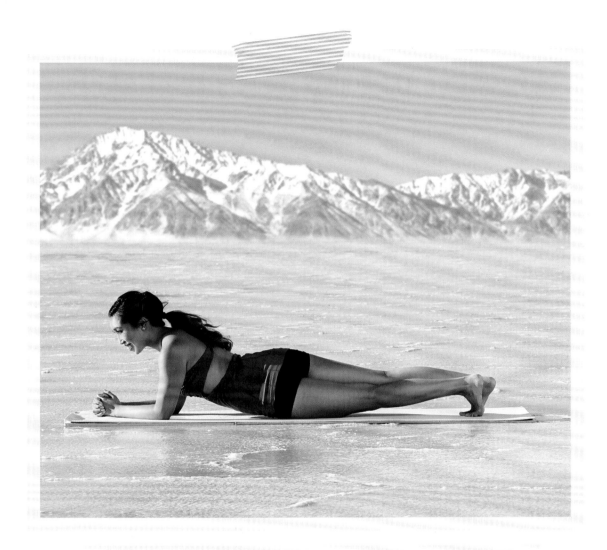

HIP TWISTS IN PLANK X 20 TAPS
WORKS: HIPS, CORE, OBLIQUES

A Place your elbows underneath you, hands clasped and legs back. Make sure your hips are up and your lower back isn't sinking. Beginners, you may get in Plank on your elbows and knees.

B Twist your hips to tap your left hip down to the mat, then tap your right hip down.

WORKOUT #2: HOT BUNS

Mmm! Nothing's better than hot buns during the winter. Feel the burn in your backside during the Bridge Circle, and especially the Fire Hydrant—laugh it out, it's a fun move.

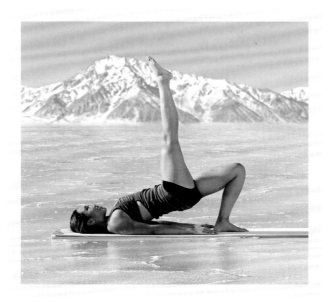

Feeling Down in the Dumps?

If you need to cry, cry. Let that negative energy out. Then, I want you to start thinking about all the amazing things that make you who you are. I want you to start bragging about yourself and I don't want you to feel bad or arrogant for one second. Accept how amazing you are and own your talent. Nothing can bring you down because you're a strong, powerful, and unstoppable person. Onward!

BRIDGE CIRCLE X
15 CLOCKWISE, 15 COUNTERCLOCKWISE, EACH LEG
WORKS: GLUTEUS, THIGHS

A Lie on your back, hands long by your sides, then push your pelvis up into Bridge. Raise your right leg up straight into the sky, toes pointed.

B Draw small circles clockwise with your lifted leg. Once you perform 15, do 15 more counterclockwise. Don't let your butt sink!

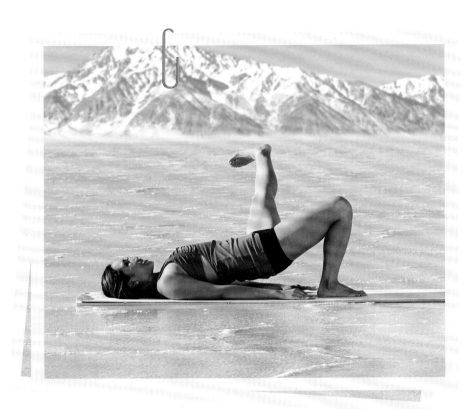

BRIDGE WIPER X 10 EACH LEG
WORKS: GLUTEUS, INNER THIGHS, OUTER THIGHS

A Lie on your back with your pelvis lifted in Bridge, arms lying by your sides. Raise your left leg straight up into the air and flex your foot. Beginners, you may lie on your back, right knee bent, left leg straight.

B Without wobbling your hips around, pretend your left leg is a windshield wiper and swing it carefully down to your left side and get as parallel as you can with the floor, inhaling. Then, on the exhale, bring it back up to start.

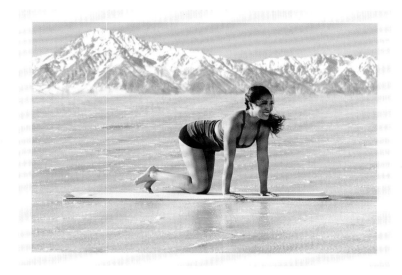

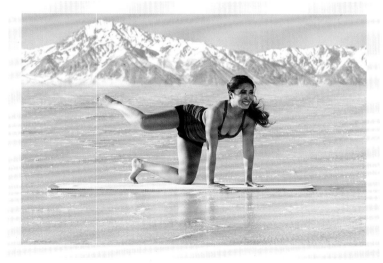

FIRE HYDRANT X 20 EACH LEG
WORKS: GLUTEUS

A Begin on all fours, hands underneath your shoulders, arms straight, and knees about hip width apart.

B Keeping your hips square to the mat and your right knee at a 90-degree angle, lift your outer thigh as high as you can, hold it, and then bring it back down without resting.

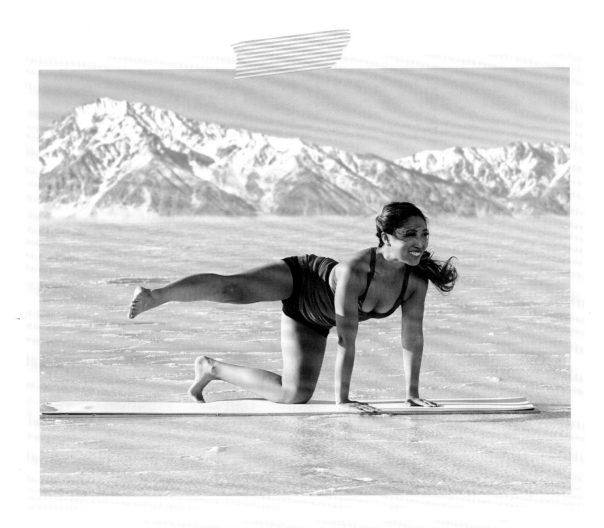

FIRE HYDRANT EXTENSION
X 15 EACH LEG
WORKS: GLUTEUS, LEGS

A Begin on all fours, hands underneath your shoulders, arms straight, and knees about hip width apart. Just as with the Fire Hydrant, lift your right knee at a 90-degree angle until your outer thigh is at hip height.

B Then point your toes and kick your right leg out to the side, bend the knee, and come back in without resting.

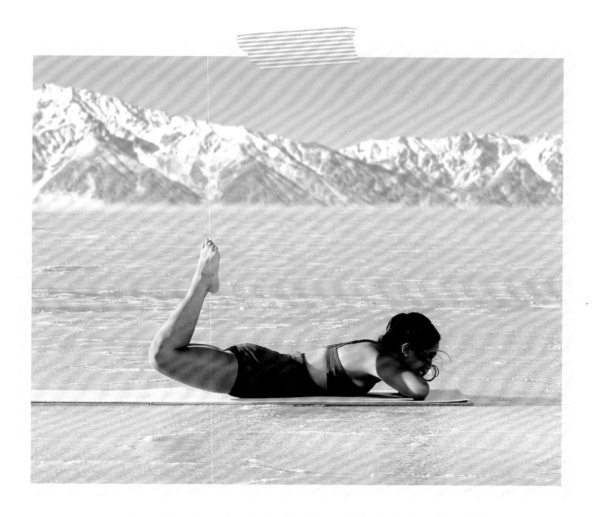

LIFTING GRASSHOPPER X 20
WORKS: GLUTEUS, LOWER BACK

A Lie on your belly with both hands underneath your chin, resting your chest on the mat. Bring your knees wide and point your feet into a diamond, toes touching.

B Squeeze your glutes and lift your knees off the mat. Try to relax your chest and put all of your energy into the lower body.

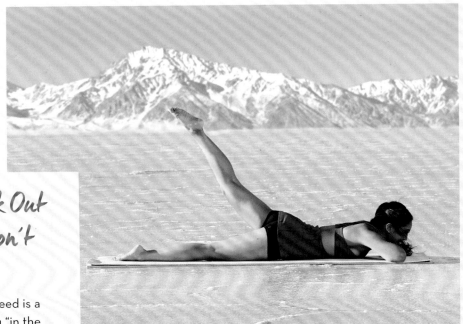

How to Work Out When You Don't Feel Like It

Sometimes all you need is a little push to get you "in the mood." Put on your favorite upbeat songs that just make you feel good! Then put on your exercise clothes and your sneakers. Write down what your workout will be. This will make you stick to it; it works miracles for me. When I want to stop, this paper acts as a personal trainer, yelling at me to keep my promise! Then, of course, just jammin' out to my favorite songs always puts me in the mood to move! I love anything pop, happy, and with some attitude.

PRONE LEG CIRCLE X 15 CLOCKWISE, 15 COUNTERCLOCKWISE, EACH LEG
WORKS: GLUTEUS, INNER THIGH, OUTER THIGH

A   Lie on your stomach with both hands resting underneath your chin and your legs long. Press your right toes into the mat for support.

B   Lift and point your left leg up as high as you can and draw circles with your toes.

WORKOUT #3: COCKTAIL DRESS LEGS

Get ready for those holiday parties and look glam whether you're going with stockings or bare, especially after you shape your legs into stunners. Burn the fat off your thighs with the cardio-intensive Plié Squat with Crisscross Jump. Then, tighten it all up with the Rockette Lunge.

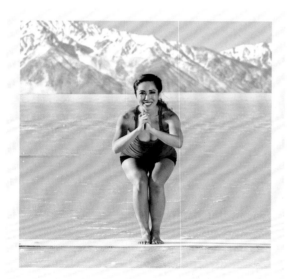 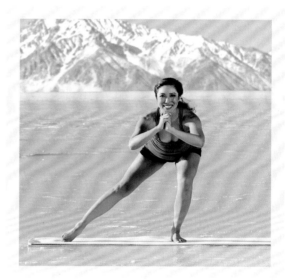

NARROW SQUAT SIDE TAP X 12 EACH LEG
WORKS: QUADS, GLUTEUS

A Stand tall on your mat, then bend into a narrow squat with your back flat, chest open, and knees together. Make sure your knees are behind your toes.

B Bring your right leg out to the side, straighten it, tap, and bring it back in the narrow squat. Stay low!

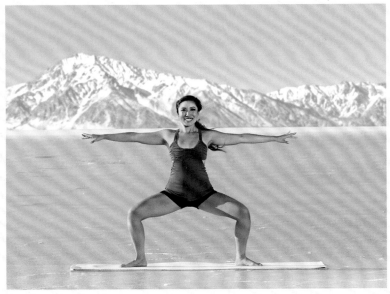

PLIÉ SQUAT WITH CRISSCROSS JUMP X 20
WORKS: THIGHS, GLUTEUS, QUADS, CARDIO

A Begin in a wide Plié Squat with your feet turned out, knees open. Pretend you're sitting your butt down and bring your arms out to the sides, fingers light.

B Pressing through the soles of your feet, push off the mat and jump high until your ankles cross. Then land lightly and immediately bounce back to that low Plié Squat. That's 1 rep!

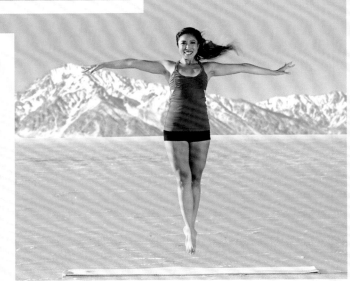

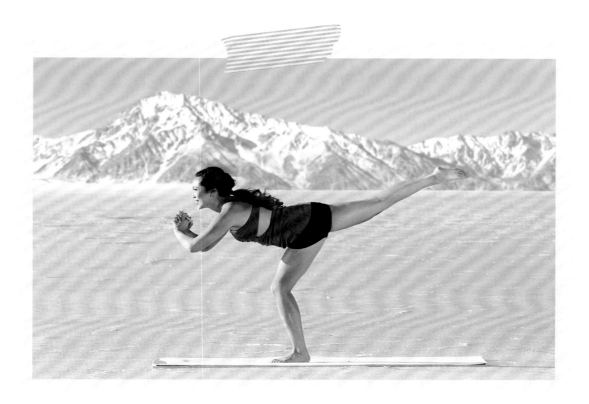

SINGLE-LEGGED T-SQUAT X
12 EACH LEG
WORKS: GLUTEUS, QUADS

A Hold your hands together and come into a narrow squat, butt back with knees behind the toes. Keeping your chest open and back tall, lift and point your right leg up and balance on your left leg.

B Straighten the left leg, then bend into a single-legged squat.

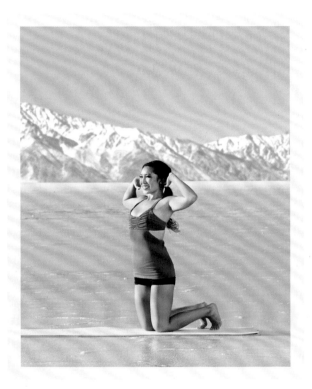 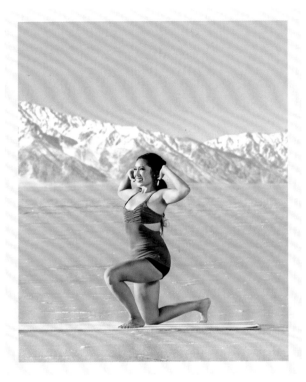

WALK THE STAIRS X 10
WORKS: QUADS, GLUTEUS, CARDIO

A Begin on your knees and place both hands behind your head, elbows wide, as if you're under arrest.

B Bring your left foot forward on the mat, followed by your right foot, then bring your left knee down, followed by your right knee. This counts as 1 rep.

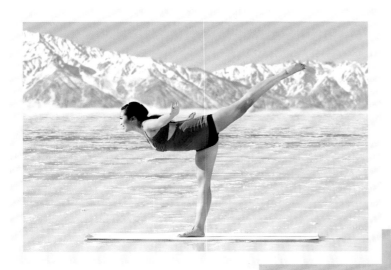

T-SEESAW POP X 10 EACH LEG
WORKS: TOTAL LOWER BODY, CARDIO

A Begin in a T position with your arms outstretched like a bird, your right leg grounded, and your left leg lifted to be in line with your back. Make sure your toes are pointed.

B Spring off of your right leg and hike your left knee into your chest, jumping while raising your arms above your head. Return back to start. That's 1 rep.

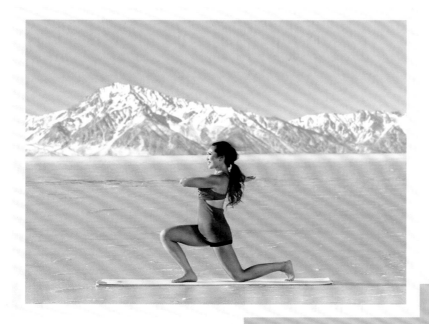

ROCKETTE LUNGE X 10 EACH SIDE
WORKS: THIGHS, GLUTEUS, QUADS

A Bring your right knee forward and your left knee down as if you're proposing. Also bring your arms out to the right side.

B In one sweeping motion, drive your left knee up into your chest and bring your arms to the left side. Return to start.

WORKOUT #4: HOLIDAY CHILL-OUT STRETCHES

Give your body a holiday of its own with these lengthening, freeing, and relaxing stretches. Feel the release of all your hard work and holiday stress while you improve your overall posture.

DANCING DOG X 15
WORKS: BACK FLEXIBILITY, TOTAL BODY AWAKENING

A Inhale and take yourself into a Down Dog position, back flat, hips up, heels stretching toward the mat, eyes on the toes.

B Exhale and bring yourself into an Up Dog position with chest lifted, hips down but not touching the mat, back arched, and hands right underneath your shoulders, arms straight. Inhale back to start. That's 1 rep.

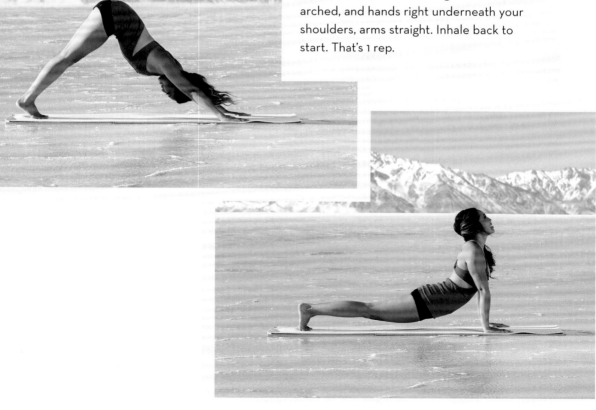

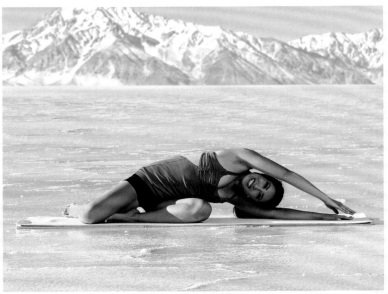

DANCING MERMAID
X 8 EACH SIDE
WORKS: BACK FLEXIBILITY, TOTAL BODY AWAKENING

A Sit tall and bring your left knee bent in front of you, your right knee bent slightly off to the side.

B Inhale and stretch over to your left side, both arms long above the head, touching the mat. Exhale and lift up to sitting, bringing your right arm into a cradle position, left arm lifted up above your head.

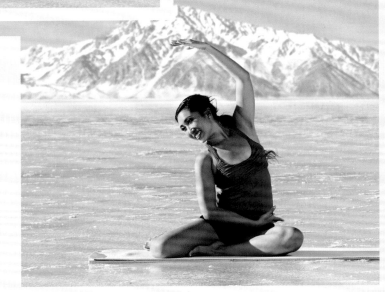

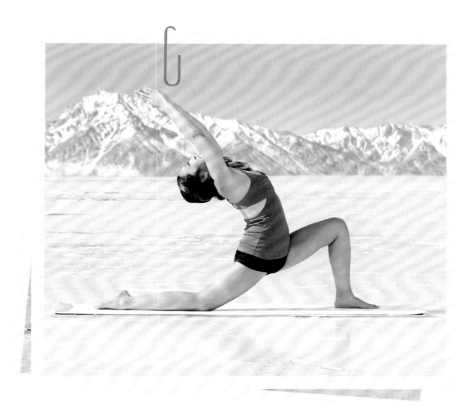

SUN LUNGE X 30 SECONDS EACH SIDE

WORKS: BACK, CHEST, GROIN

A Get into a low lunge with your left leg in front, knee up, and your right leg long behind you, knee resting on the mat.

B Bring your hands into a prayer position, palms together, and raise your arms long above your head. Then arch and stretch your spine back.

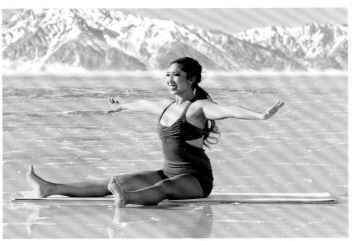

SPINE TWIST X 12
WORKS: POSTURE, BACK

A Sit comfortably on your bottom with your spine super tall, shoulders relaxed, crown of the head still enough to balance a tiara. Bring your arms out to the side like airplane wings.

B Exhale and bring your left fingers to your right toes, looking back at your right hand. Then inhale and inflate your spine tall. This is 1 rep.

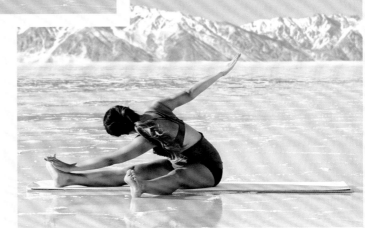

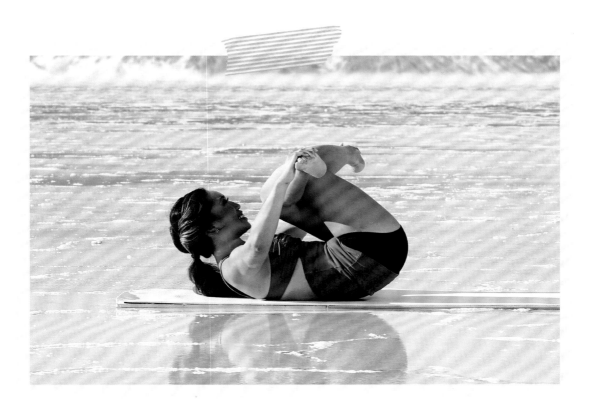

CRISSCROSS BUTT
X 30 SECONDS EACH SIDE
WORKS: GLUTEUS

A Lie on your back with your right knee crossed over your left knee. Hold on to the tops of your feet and pull your toes toward your shoulders. Hold for 30 seconds, then repeat on the other side.

No-Time Quickie Workout!

There are days when a full-length gym session just isn't going to happen. It's okay. Whatever you can get in is good! Here's a total body workout you should do if you've got about 10 minutes to spare:

1. Single-Legged T-Squat x 12 each leg (page 213)
2. Hip Twisting Butt-Up x 12 (page 154)
3. Push-up to Side Plank x 12 (page 168)
4. Eagle Crunch x 15 (page 48)
5. Star Abs x 15 (page 97)

Repeat 3 times.

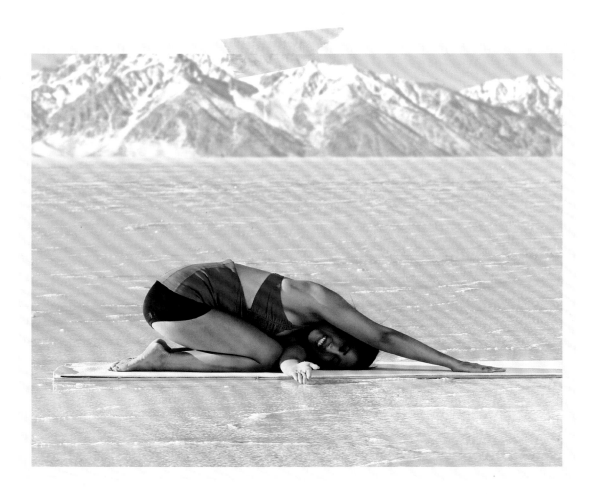

CHILD THREADING THE NEEDLE X 30 SECONDS EACH SIDE
WORKS: UPPER BACK

A Get into Child's Pose with your chest resting on your knees and both arms surrendered in front of you, head relaxed.

B Thread your left arm underneath your right arm, palm open. Press your left shoulder into your left knee and your elbow into the mat.

WORKOUT #5: PRE-PARTY TONE-UP

Crank up the volume and prepare yourself for a total body party! Do the Cha-Cha-Cha Abs to tighten up your abs, the Single-Legged Limbo Push-up for toned arms and a tight core, and the empowering Airplane move that's sure to warrant applause.

PLANK TAP-OUT X 8
WORKS: CORE, SHOULDERS

A Begin in Plank with your hands underneath your shoulders, arm straight, body long, feet hip width apart. Tap your left shoulder with your right hand and move that hand one hand-length back from where it was. Then tap your right shoulder with your left hand and move that hand one hand-length back from where it was. Do this until your hands touch your toes.

B Repeat the alternating shoulder-tapping, hand-moving motions as you walk your way back out to Plank. One trip in and out counts as 1 rep!

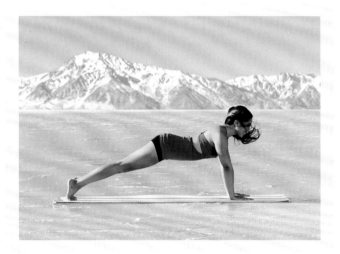

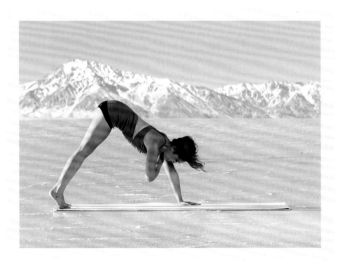

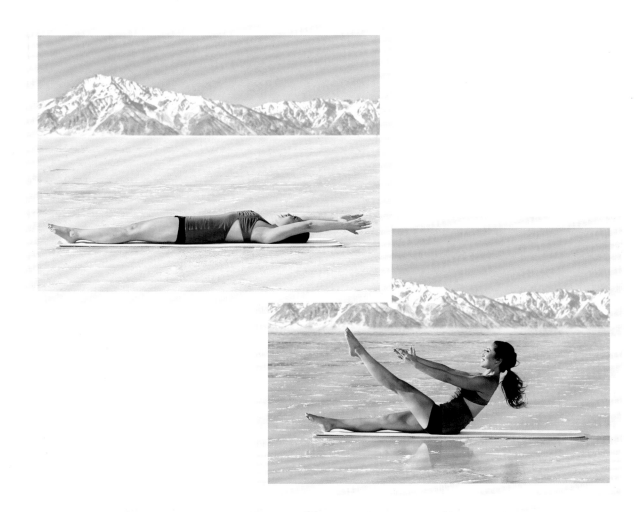

SINGLE-LEGGED JACKKNIFE X 16
WORKS: ABS, QUADS

A Lie down, back flat on the mat, legs long in front of you, arms long behind you.

B Exhale and raise your left leg up to a diagonal as you peel your back off the mat and sit up with your arms stretched forward. Then inhale and slowly lay your back down on the mat, and return the leg to the floor. Alternate legs. That's 1 rep.

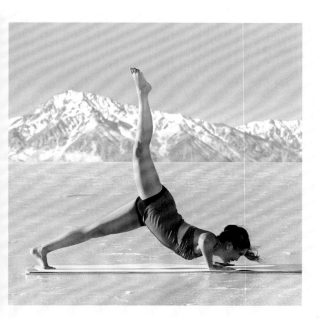

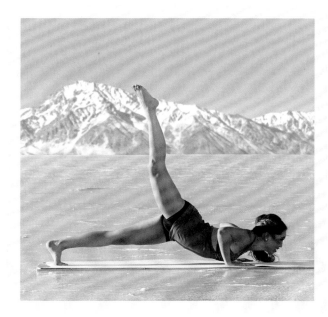

SINGLE-LEGGED LIMBO
PUSH-UP X 5 EACH LEG
WORKS: TOTAL UPPER BODY

A Begin in a Down Dog position, heels stretched toward the mat, back flat, eyes on the toes, hips up, palms flat. Then lift your right leg off the mat to get into a single-legged Down Dog position. Beginners, you may keep both feet on the mat.

B Pretend there is a limbo bar that is positioned a couple feet off the mat. Graze your chest against the floor in a push-up position and try to pull your whole body underneath the imaginary bar without touching it until you end up in a single-legged Up Dog. Push back to start. That's 1 rep.

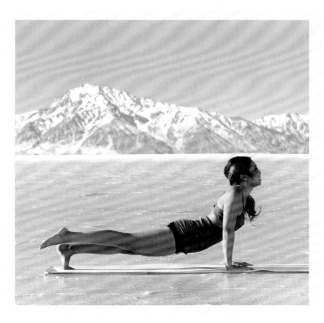

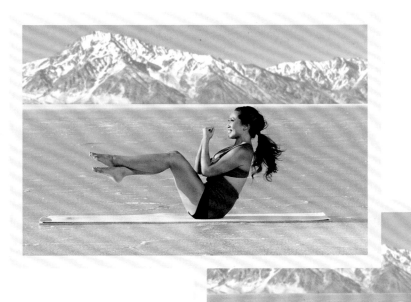

BOXER X 20
WORKS: QUADS, CORE, ARMS

A Begin by balancing on your tailbone, knees bent and lifted off the mat, ankles crossed, toes pointed. Your hands should be in fists in a "ready to fight" boxer position, covering your face for protection.

B Exhale and powerfully punch your right arm to the left side and extend your legs out. Inhale and bring everything back in. Then punch your left arm to the right with the leg extension. Each punch is 1 rep.

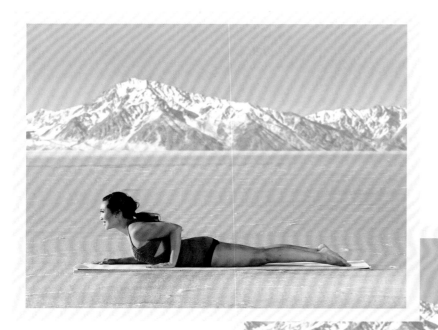

STAGGERED TRICEP PRESS
X 15 EACH SIDE
WORKS: TRICEPS, CHEST

A Lie on your belly with both hands by your shoulders, elbows into your rib cage. Then slide your right arm forward toward the edge of your mat.

B Exhale and lift your chest off the mat until your right arm is straight. Inhale and return to start.

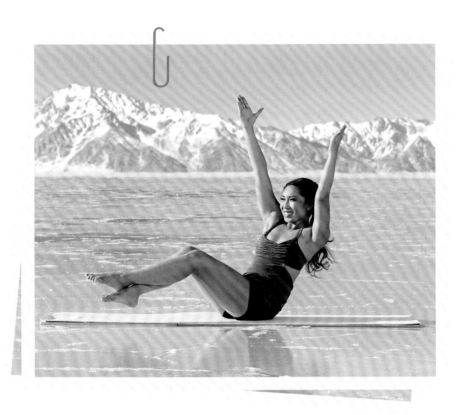

CHA-CHA-CHA ABS X 15
WORKS: TRANSVERSE ABS

A Sit on your tailbone with your knees together and facing upward, feet off the
floor. Raise your arms so that they are extended long above your head. Make
sure to lengthen your neck and relax your shoulders away from your ears.

B Drop your left shoulder farther down and pull with your left transverse
abdominal. Then drop your right shoulder down and pull with your right
transverse abdominal. One more drop with the left shoulder again. Your arms
should be straight the whole time. Each shoulder drop is like a shimmy. There are 3
shimmies in one Cha-Cha-Cha Ab and that counts as 1 rep.

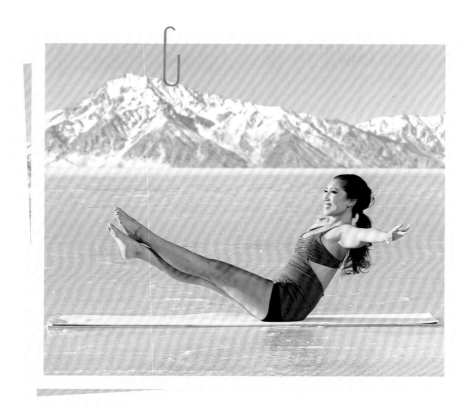

AIRPLANE FOR 15-SECOND HOLD X 3
WORKS: CORE, QUADS

A Balance on your tailbone and cross your ankles, back tall.

B Open up your arms and push your feet forward until your legs are long and straight. Hold right here! This is an extremely challenging position, especially for those with lower back issues. To modify, curl your back into a Pilates C-Curve to protect your back and keep your legs long in front of you on the mat.

A Note from Cassey

Why Are You Eating When You're Not Hungry?

You walk to the fridge, open the door, and just stare, mesmerized. There's something so comforting about gazing into the bright glow that lights your food with what seems like a holy aura. Then you reach in and grab something to eat. Somehow, the food fills a need at the moment. Somehow, it's the only thing that seems to understand you, right then and there.

You may not be hungry. In fact, most of the time you're not. You're just bored, or sad, or just trying to avoid doing something you don't want to do. Trust me, there's been many a time when I've started to get fidgety from not wanting to work or study, and then I head to the kitchen to stuff my face with some snacks as a momentary distraction.

This is what I'm usually thinking, "The sweet and salty crunch of this honey-mustard pretzel bite is hypnotic. It feels so good. I can't stop. Oops, the whole bag is gone. Oh, wait, what's that? Let's try some of this leftover pizza. Mmm. I'm not full yet. Let's see if this french vanilla ice cream will do it. Ah, perfect."

Food is comfort. Food reminds us of Mom. Of home. Of childhood. Being fed and feeling full are nice things. So it's only natural to want to use food as a way to fill some void or serve as a distraction (boxes of chocolates after a breakup, anyone?!). However, you can't let food be the answer to everything. This is how the calories add up and the weight layers on your body.

To stop the emotional eating, take a moment and ask yourself if you're actually really hungry. Not sure? It's okay. So grab a glass of water and drink that while you keep thinking. If your body begins to yearn for something more, grab a fruit or a healthy snack, like carrots and hummus, and think some more. Be in a peaceful place. Are you trying to get away from a situation that doesn't feel good? Did something happen today that made you feel sad? Try to find a friend and talk it out. That's the best way to release negative energy and clear the emotional toxins that are forcing you to seek food as an answer.

All you really want is to be balanced again, to fill that void. It's a hunger to feel whole again, not a hunger for food. Simply be conscious of the fact that you may be dealing with an emotional issue, not a calorie deficiency. Once you realize that, you will be in control of your eating habits.

Good luck, guys! I know you can do this.

♡ Cassey

WINTER EATS

Winter is a great test of our culinary creativity! A lot of the fun fruits and veggies aren't in season, so it's important to know what *is* available in a way that continues to excite you. For instance, spaghetti squash, a hard winter squash, is a perfect base for your imagination; it absorbs flavor easily and is a lot like real spaghetti, but it's cleaner and healthier. I suggest serving it with marinara, but feel free to mix the spaghetti-like strands with any vegetables and light, veggie-forward sauces your heart desires!

Remember the season: invite Santa on your holiday journey and leave him the Peppermint Brownies (page 240) instead of sugar cookies! Organize a cookie exchange with friends, but encourage healthier cookies and hand out prizes for "Best Taste," "Most Creative," and "Better Luck Next Time." You will all have a good laugh, I promise.

WINTER'S IN-SEASON GROCERY LIST

Vegetables
Acorn squash
Belgian endive
Brussels
    sprouts
Butternut
    squash
cauliflower
collard greens

jicama
kale
sweet potatoes

Fruits
clementines
dates
grapefruit
kiwi

oranges
passion fruit
pears
pineapple
pomegranate
tangerines

Microwave Minute Pumpkin Muffin

INGREDIENTS

- 1 large egg
- 2 tablespoons canned pumpkin puree
- 1 teaspoon ground cinnamon
- Pinch of ground nutmeg
- ½ teaspoon vanilla extract
- 2 teaspoons stevia
- ¼ cup quick-cooking oats
- 1 tablespoon plain soy or unsweetened almond milk (optional)

DIRECTIONS

In a coffee mug, whip together the egg, pumpkin puree, cinnamon, nutmeg, vanilla, and stevia. Fold in the oats. If desired, stir in a little soy or almond milk to reach pourable consistency.

Place the mug in the microwave and heat on high for 1 minute (keep an eye on it; the muffin can rise quickly). Test to see if the top is firm; if not, place back in the microwave and heat for an additional 30 seconds.

Let cool for 1 minute, then turn out of the mug onto a plate to serve.

160 calories, 6g fat, 16g carbs, 9g protein, 2g sugar

MAKES 1 MUFFIN

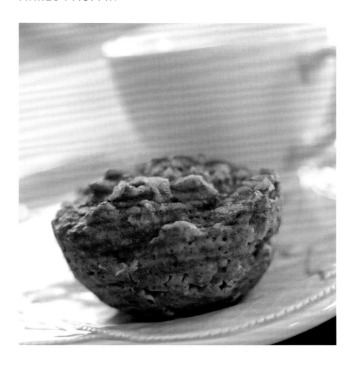

Wonder Waffles

INGREDIENTS

6 tablespoons water

2 tablespoons ground flaxseed

Cooking spray

1¾ cups whole wheat flour

½ teaspoon salt

2 teaspoons baking soda

3 teaspoons stevia

¾ cups old-fashioned rolled oats

2 cups unsweetened vanilla soy or almond milk

⅓ cup melted coconut oil

1 teaspoon vanilla extract

DIRECTIONS

Whisk the water and flaxseed in a small bowl and let sit for 10 minutes.

Heat and lightly coat a waffle iron with cooking spray.

Stir the flour, salt, baking soda, stevia, and oats together in a bowl. In a separate bowl, combine the flaxseed mixture with the soy milk, coconut oil, and vanilla.

Place the wet and dry ingredients in a blender and blend until well combined. Pour one-fourth of the batter into a heated, lightly greased waffle iron. Cook the waffle according to the manufacturer's instructions for approximately 4 to 5 minutes or until the waffle iron alerts that the waffle is ready. Repeat with the remaining batter.

(for 1 waffle): 279 calories, 15g fat, 33g carbs, 7g protein, .2g sugar

MAKES 4 WAFFLES

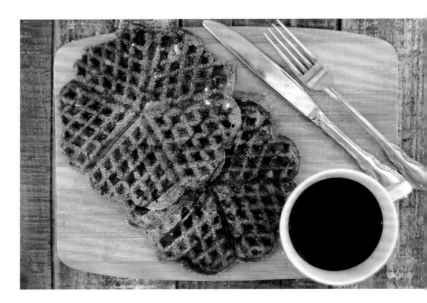

Kale and White Bean Soup

INGREDIENTS

- 2 teaspoons olive oil
- ⅓ onion, chopped
- 1 garlic clove, crushed
- 1 carrot, chopped
- 1 teaspoon dried thyme
- 1 teaspoon dried oregano
- 1 (14.5 oz.) can cannellini beans, drained and rinsed
- 3 cups vegetable stock
- 3 cups chopped fresh kale, thick stems removed
- Salt and pepper to taste

DIRECTIONS

In a medium saucepan, heat the olive oil over medium-high heat. Add the onion, garlic, carrot, thyme, and oregano and cook for 5 minutes, stirring occasionally, until the vegetables are soft.

Add ¼ cup of the beans and smash them with the back of a wooden spoon. Add the stock and bring to a boil. Stir in the kale, the remaining beans, and salt and pepper. Lower the heat and simmer for approximately 10 minutes.

(for 1 serving): 207 calories, 3g fat, 36g carbs, 11g protein, 3g sugar

SERVES 4

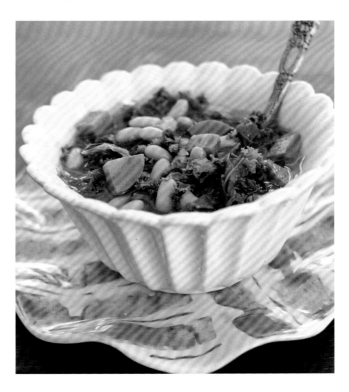

Loaded Baked Potato

INGREDIENTS

- 1 medium sweet potato
- 1 (4-ounce) chicken cutlet, cooked and shredded
- 1 cup trimmed fresh spinach
- ¼ cup canned black beans, rinsed and drained
- ¼ cup favorite salsa
- 2 tablespoons 2% Greek yogurt

DIRECTIONS

Puncture the sweet potato with a fork in four or five places. Place on a microwave-safe dish and microwave on high for 5 to 8 minutes.

Combine the chicken, spinach, and beans in a small saucepan and simmer over low-medium heat.

Cut the sweet potato lengthwise, then stuff the split with the chicken mixture. Top with salsa and a dollop of Greek yogurt, and serve.

337 calories, 5g fat, 40g carbs, 35g protein, 11g sugar

SERVES 1

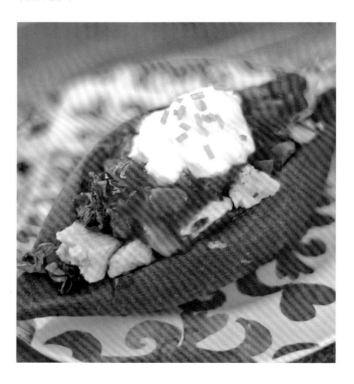

Spaghetti Squash Supper

INGREDIENTS

½ medium spaghetti squash, halved, seeds removed

1 cup cherry tomatoes, sliced in half

2 teaspoons olive oil

1 garlic clove, crushed

4 ounces ground turkey

2 tablespoons chopped fresh parsley

Salt and pepper to taste

DIRECTIONS

Preheat the oven to 375°F.

Place the spaghetti squash cut side down in a small baking pan. Pour about 1 cup of water into the pan and roast the squash for 35 to 40 minutes, until tender. Set aside to cool briefly.

While the squash bakes, toss the tomatoes with the olive oil and garlic in a medium ovenproof bowl and roast for 10 minutes.

Add the turkey to the tomatoes and roast for an additional 15 minutes. Stir in the parsley, salt, and pepper.

Using tongs to hold the squash, use a fork to scrape out the inside horizontally, making "spaghetti." Toss the spaghetti squash with the tomato-turkey mixture and serve.

330 calories, 13g fat, 26g carbs, 28g protein, 10g sugar

SERVES 1

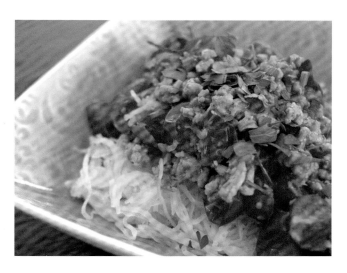

Veggie Sloppy Joe

INGREDIENTS

- 1 teaspoon olive oil
- ¼ cup chopped green bell pepper
- ½ garlic clove, minced
- ½ cup tomato sauce
- Pinch of red pepper flakes
- ¼ cup vegan chorizo or meatless crumble
- ½ cup grated zucchini
- 1 whole wheat bun
- ½ cup shredded cabbage, lettuce, or other leafy vegetable

DIRECTIONS

Heat the olive oil in a medium nonstick saucepan over medium heat. Add the green pepper and garlic and sauté for 5 to 6 minutes, stirring occasionally, until soft.

Add the tomato sauce, red pepper flakes, chorizo, and zucchini. Lower the heat and simmer for 5 minutes, until flavors blend.

Open the bun and pour the tomato mixture over the tops. Top with cabbage, lettuce, or other veggies.

327 calories, 14g fat, 42g carbs, 15g protein, 11g sugar

SERVES 1

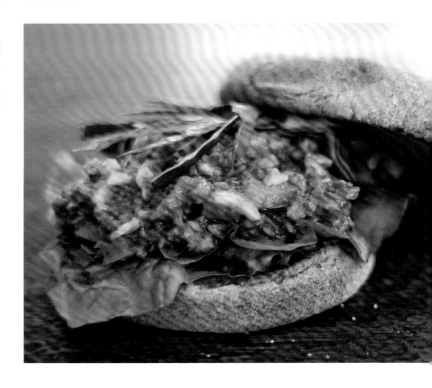

Gingerbread Fonuts

INGREDIENTS

FONUTS

Cooking spray

1¼ cups almond meal

¼ teaspoon salt

¼ teaspoon baking soda

1 teaspoon ground ginger

1 teaspoon ground cinnamon

⅓ teaspoon ground allspice

Pinch of ground cloves

3 large eggs, lightly beaten

2 tablespoons honey

¼ cup melted coconut oil

½ teaspoon vanilla extract

FROSTING

½ medium banana

2 tablespoons Tofutti cream cheese

Assorted toppings: cinnamon, chopped walnuts, shaved chocolate

DIRECTIONS

Make the fonuts: Coat a nonstick mini donut maker with cooking spray. In a large mixing bowl, combine the almond meal, salt, baking soda, ginger, cinnamon, allspice, cloves, eggs, honey, coconut oil, and vanilla. Pour 2 to 3 tablespoons of the batter into each donut cup and cook until the donut maker signals they are done, or until a toothpick inserted in the center comes out clean. Unmold and cool on a rack.

Make the frosting: Mash the banana with the back of a wooden spoon or a fork. Combine with the cream cheese in a food processor or blender until smooth, adding water to thin, if necessary.

Dip the fonuts into the frosting and sprinkle with your favorite toppings.

(for 2 fonuts): 139 calories, 12g fat, 5g carbs, 4g protein, 2g sugar

MAKES 24 FONUTS

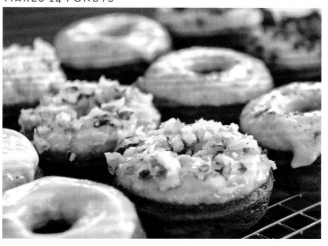

Peppermint Brownies

INGREDIENTS

Cooking spray

6 tablespoons water

2 tablespoons ground flaxseed

1 (15-ounce) can black beans, well rinsed and drained

3 tablespoons melted coconut oil

¾ cup unsweetened cocoa powder

⅓ cup agave nectar

1½ teaspoons baking powder

1 teaspoon vanilla extract

⅛ teaspoon peppermint extract

DIRECTIONS

Preheat the oven to 350°F. Coat an 8-inch square baking pan with cooking spray.

Whisk the water and flaxseed in a small bowl. Let sit for 10 minutes.

Combine the flaxseed mixture, the beans, coconut oil, cocoa powder, agave nectar, baking powder, and extracts in a food processor and blend until smooth.

Pour the batter into the baking pan and bake the brownies for 20 to 25 minutes, or until a toothpick comes out moist and with some crumbs. Let cool for 30 minutes, then score the top into 12 pieces and remove from the pan.

(for 1 brownie): 120 calories, 5g fat, 19g carbs, 15g protein, 11g sugar

MAKES 12 BROWNIES

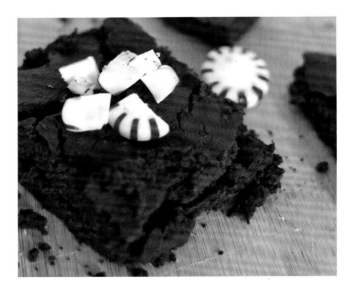

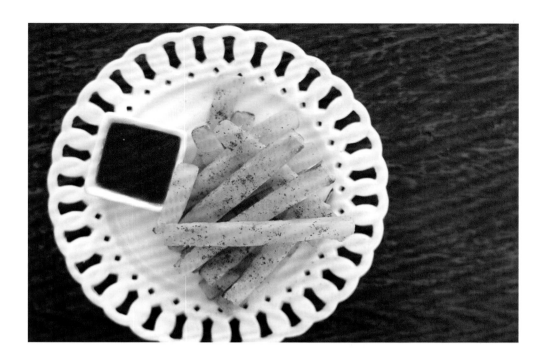

Butternut Squash Fries

INGREDIENTS

Cooking spray

½ medium butternut squash, peeled, seeded, and cut into julienne

Olive oil spray

Assorted seasonings (optional): salt and pepper, stevia, ground cinnamon, chili powder

DIRECTIONS

Preheat the oven to 450°F. Coat a baking sheet with cooking spray.

In a bowl, spray the squash with oil and toss with seasonings of your choice, if desired.

Arrange the squash pieces in a single layer on the baking sheet and bake for 16 to 19 minutes, until the fries are crisp.

(for 5-7 fries): 61 calories, .2g fat, 16g carbs, 1g protein, 0g sugar

SERVES 4

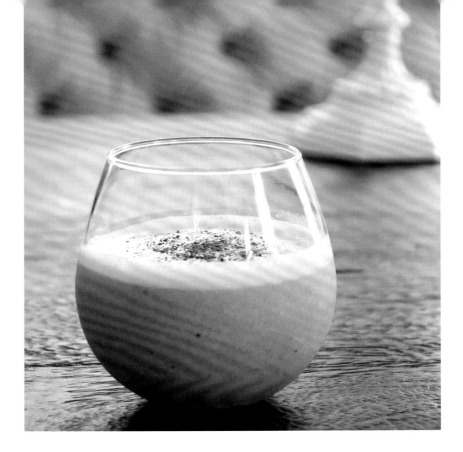

Egg Nog Smoothie

INGREDIENTS

½ cup unsweetened vanilla almond milk

1 frozen medium banana

Pinch of ground nutmeg

Pinch of ground cloves

¼ teaspoon ground cinnamon

DIRECTIONS

Place all the ingredients in a blender and process until smooth. Pour into a tall glass and serve.

135 calories, 3g fat, 28g carbs, 2.3g protein, 15g sugar

MAKES 1

A Note from Cassey

Stop feeling guilty. **Stop it!** The holidays are a time to enjoy food, family, and friends. It's not every day that you get to taste fabulous home-cooked meals, so quit thinking so much about calories and fat, and just live. Food is such a big part of our culture; not only does it nourish our bodies, but it also brings people together in a celebratory environment. Let food make you happy.

It's totally okay to have a yolo meal once in a while to speed up your metabolism and keep you sane! If you're going to indulge, then indulge 100 percent. Enjoy the experience because feeling bad about it won't change the situation.

The best way to deal with the holidays, the overabundance of food, and your waistline is to **indulge smartly**. Yes, you can have the pie and the buttered potatoes—but only after you've filled your plate with vegetables and lean protein. And if you're still afraid that you won't be able to resist, then plan for success. Eat healthy before the party to "pre-fill" yourself. Bring a salad for the potluck. Do some extra cardio the next day.

Remember, you are not doomed! You are always in control of your own success. Don't put yourself in the position of "victim" when you **know** you can determine your own destiny.

Eat well and laugh a lot! Save a slice of cake for me. :)

♡ Cassey

Winter Fast-Track Meal Plan

SUNDAY	MONDAY	TUESDAY	WEDNESDAY
Breakfast Microwave Minute Pumpkin Muffin (page 233)	**Breakfast** High-fiber cereal with unsweetened almond milk and 2 tablespoons ground flaxseed	**Breakfast** Smooth almond oatmeal: 1 cup cooked oatmeal, 1 tablespoon almond butter, and 1 teaspoon agave nectar	**Breakfast** High-fiber cereal with unsweetened almond milk and 2 tablespoons ground flaxseed
Snack Peppermint Brownies (page 240)	**Snack** Egg Nog Smoothie (page 242)	**Snack** Peppermint Brownies (page 240)	**Snack** 2 rice crackers with 1 low-fat string cheese
Lunch Egg(less) Salad Sandwich (page 136)	**Lunch** Kale and White Bean Soup (page 235)	**Lunch** Loaded Baked Potato (page 236)	**Lunch** Chickpea salad: ½ cup cooked quinoa, ⅓ cup canned chickpeas, 1 chopped ripe tomato, 1 chopped Persian cucumber, and 1 cup chopped fresh spinach, tossed with 1 tablespoon lemon juice, 1 teaspoon Dijon mustard, and 1 tablespoon chopped fresh parsley
Snack 1 pear, 10 almonds	**Snack** Peppermint Brownies (page 240)	**Snack** 1 small banana, 1 tablespoon almond butter	**Snack** ½ avocado drizzled with lemon juice
Dinner Turkey plate: 1 (4-ounce) cooked turkey cutlet and 1 cup roasted Brussels sprouts (cut in half, tossed with extra-virgin olive oil spray, and roasted at 400°F for 20 minutes)	**Dinner** Chickpea curry: ⅓ cup chickpeas (garbanzo beans) sautéed with ⅓ cup chopped tofu, ½ cup chopped cauliflower, 2 cups chopped kale, 1 teaspoon curry powder, and 2 tablespoons water	**Dinner** Chicken and veggies: 1 (4-ounce) roasted chicken cutlet, 2 cups steamed veggies (broccoli, cauliflower, kale), and 1 medium sweet potato	**Dinner** Spaghetti Squash Supper (page 237)

Recipes with page references are included in this book; others are quick and easy to put together in a flash!

THURSDAY	FRIDAY	SATURDAY
Breakfast Breakfast smoothie: ½ pear, 1 kiwi, ½ frozen banana, 1 cup chopped spinach, 1 scoop protein powder, and water to thin to desired consistency	**Breakfast** Crunchy almond oatmeal: 1 cup cooked oatmeal, 5 chopped almonds, 1 teaspoon ground cinnamon, 1 teaspoon stevia	**Breakfast** Wonder Waffles (page 234)
Snack 3 slices low-sodium turkey, 1 apple	**Snack** Peppermint Brownies (page 240)	**Snack** 1 cup cauliflower florets, ¼ cup hummus
Lunch Kale and White Bean Soup (page 235)	**Lunch** BLT: 2 slices of sprouted grain toast, 2 slices turkey bacon, 1 sliced ripe tomato, handful of mixed greens	**Lunch** Muffin pizza: whole wheat English muffin topped with ¼ cup tomato sauce, ¼ cup steamed chopped broccoli, 4 ounces low-sodium turkey slices, and sprinkling of Parmesan cheese
Snack Plain 2% Greek yogurt	**Snack** 1 grapefruit, 10 cashews	**Snack** 1 small apple, 1 tablespoon almond butter
Dinner Fiesta chicken: 1 (4-ounce) cooked chicken cutlet served with guacamole (½ avocado, 1 chopped tomato, 1 tablespoon fresh cilantro, 2 teaspoons lime juice, 1 teaspoon chopped jalapeño), served with 2 cups mixed greens	**Dinner** Cauliflower mash: 2 cups steamed cauliflower, blended in a food processor until smooth with 2 tablespoons 2% Greek yogurt, served with 1 (4-ounce) cooked turkey or chicken cutlet and 2 cups steamed kale	**Dinner** Veggie Sloppy Joe (page 238)

We did it, guys!

I hope you enjoyed spending the seasons traveling and working out with me in my first book! You now have a treasure chest of moves to pick from when you're exercising for yourself or when you're teaching your friends.

Practice as much as you can not only to get lean but also to get stronger and more graceful with your movements. I want you to be able to control your body the way you want it to move. I also want to see you do things you never thought you were capable of doing! It's in you, I promise.

Also, though the routines in this book are aimed at helping you sculpt a beautiful body, remember that you already *are* beautiful—don't let the number between your feet define your self-worth. It's not about the vanity. Look beyond the superficial. Let these empowering exercises ignite your fire for living purposefully and passionately. Finding peace within yourself is the enlightened state of happiness that you embrace as you keep progressing. This is the best success one can ask for.

I love you so much!

♡ Cassey

ACKNOWLEDGMENTS

You know how when you're a kid and you tell your friends, "One day I'm going to write a book about this!" For many of us, it's a saying that we toss around in laughter. I never thought that one day I'd *actually* have the opportunity to publish a book with one of the top publishing companies in America. I am beyond grateful to everyone who has shaped my experiences to help lead me to the path I am on.

Thank you to all my teachers in school for constantly encouraging me to be a better writer, which turned me into a blogger . . . which turned me into an author.

A special shout-out to Dr. Crain for your belief in me, even as a confused college student. I graduated from Whittier College with a degree in biology, but also with a friendship that I can hold forever.

Thank you to Evelia Burnett who gave me my first ever Pilates job!

Thank you to all the Pilates students I have ever taught! Seeing your sweaty smiling faces in class is what I *live* for.

Thank you to Stephanie Knapp and Heather Jackson of Random House for giving me the opportunity to share my expertise with the world.

Thank you, David Kim, for traveling all over the United States with me to shoot the gorgeous photos for this book. I'll never forget the hopeless expressions on our faces after we climbed that crazy mountain in Utah, with all our camera gear in the bitter cold, only to find that there were no more wildflowers by the lake. Or the time I was floating on a yoga mat in the middle of the Salt Flats. Good times!

Thank you to Danielle Bernabe for cooking and testing all the recipes in this book with me. Our hero burger is not to be messed with.

Thank you to my pals at YouTube who gave me the opportunity to upload my first workout video back in 2009. Your constant work to promote your creators' content is turning the traditional entertainment world upside down. I'm so happy to be a part of our Wild West.

Thank you to Will Hobbs for embracing me with your kindness, intellect, and big visions for Blogilates! Remember when you first asked me if I wanted to write a book and I was like "what?" Well, thanks for asking. We're making so many cool things happen together.

Thank you to my baby sister, Jackelyn, for always encouraging me to live my dreams. Your vibrancy, positivity, and leadership always push me to work harder and live the life I want. We Ho sisters are unstoppable. I love you, Am!

Thank you to my mom for always, always, always believing in me. Your enthusiastic support of all of my endeavors while growing up (sewing all the Halloween costumes and prom dresses I designed, working late with me to bake sweets for my first fully functioning high school cookie business, COOPLEX, helping me make the first oGorgeous bag samples, reading my YouTube comments) and now with Blogilates has helped me become a fearless entrepreneur. Your love makes me ever more resilient. Thank you. I love you so much, Mommy!

Thank you to my dad for being you. Sometimes our fires clash but only to mold us to who we're meant to be. Even though we've had our rough patches, our journey really has come full circle. I couldn't be happier than to know that you're proud of me and that we can work together to make big things happen. Thank you. I love you.

And thank you to Sam. Can you believe where we started and where we are now?! So much hard work, but honestly, what else would we be doing with our time? Dreams really can come true, and I am so happy that I am living them with you. Love you, Woodge.

WHERE TO FIND ME!

YOUTUBE: free workouts every single week!
YOUTUBE.COM/BLOGILATES

MY BLOG: for daily updates on my new video workouts and best healthy recipes
BLOGILATES.COM

THE BLOGILATES APP:
available on iPhone and Android

FACEBOOK: LIKE ME ON FACEBOOK.COM/BLOGILATES

TWITTER: TWEET ME AT @BLOGILATES

INSTAGRAM: FOLLOW ME AT @BLOGILATES

MY ACTIVEWEAR COLLECTION: BODYPOPACTIVE.COM

REFERENCES

"The Acute Effects of Exercise on Mood State." See https://ulib.derby.ac.uk/ecdu/CourseRes/dbs/currissu/Yeung_R.pdf.

Dillman, Erika. *The Little Pilates Book*. New York: Warner Books, 2001.

Giampapa, Vincent, Ronald Pero, and Marcia Zimmerman. *The Anti-Aging Solution*. Hoboken, NJ: John Wiley, 2004.

Gleick, James. *Chaos: Making a New Science*. New York: Penguin, 1987.

Griffith, H. Winter. *Minerals, Supplements, & Vitamins: The Essential Guide*. Tucson, AZ: Fisher, 2000.

"History of Joseph Pilates." *Pilates Technique*. PilatesTechnique. www.josephpilates.com/joomla/history-of-joseph-pilatesa-little-about-the-man-behind-it-all.html.

Marrone, Margo. *The Organic Pharmacy*. New York: Duncan Baird, 2009.

Pronk, N. P., S. F. Crouse, and J. J. Rohack. "Maximal Exercise and Acute Mood Response in Women." *Physiology and Behavior,* 57 (1995): 1–4.

Stanway, Penny. *The Miracle of Lemons: Practical Tips for Health, Home, and Beauty*. London: Watkins, 1988.

Tannis, Allison. *Feed Your Skin, Starve Your Wrinkles*. Rockport, MA: Fair Winds Press, 2009.

"Water: How Much Should You Drink Every Day?" Mayo Foundation for Medical Education and Research. www.mayoclinic.org/healthy-living/nutrition-and-healthy-eating/in-depth/water/art-20044256.

RECIPE INDEX

EXERCISE INDEX

Note: (W) denotes workouts; exercises are indexed under their names.

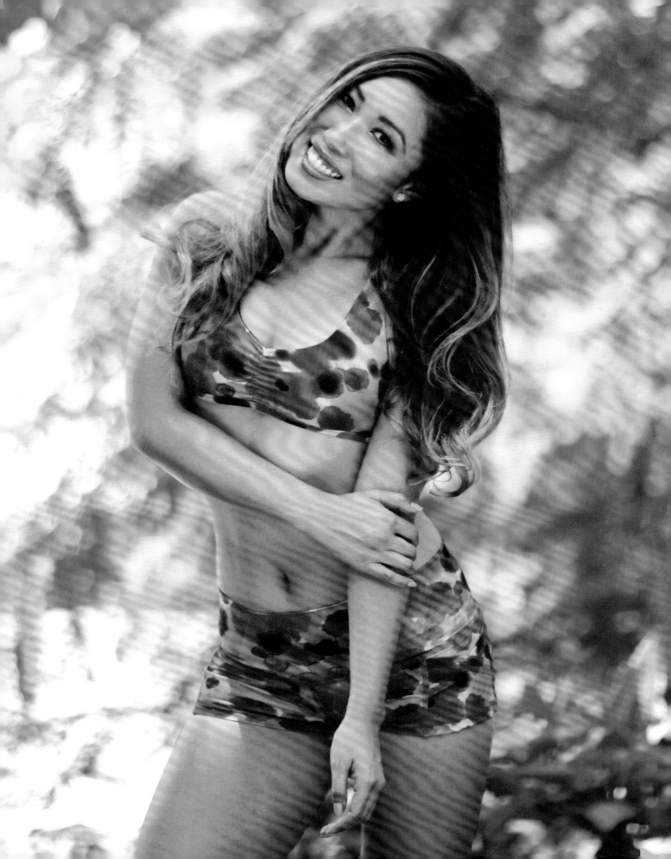